HASHIMOTO'S COOKBOOK GLUTTEN FREE

An effortless guide for Managing Hashimoto's Thyroiditis with Delicious, Nutrient-Rich Recipes

Dr. Kelly Haaland

Dear Valued Reader,

First and foremost, we want to extend our heartfelt thanks for choosing our cookbook. Your trust in our culinary collection means the world to us. If our cookbook has brought joy to your kitchen and table, we'd be thrilled to hear about your experiences in an Amazon review. On the flip side, if you stumble upon any hiccups while exploring our recipes, don't hesitate to get in touch at **kellyhaaland2@gmail.com** We're here to support your cooking journey every step of the way.

Warmest regards,

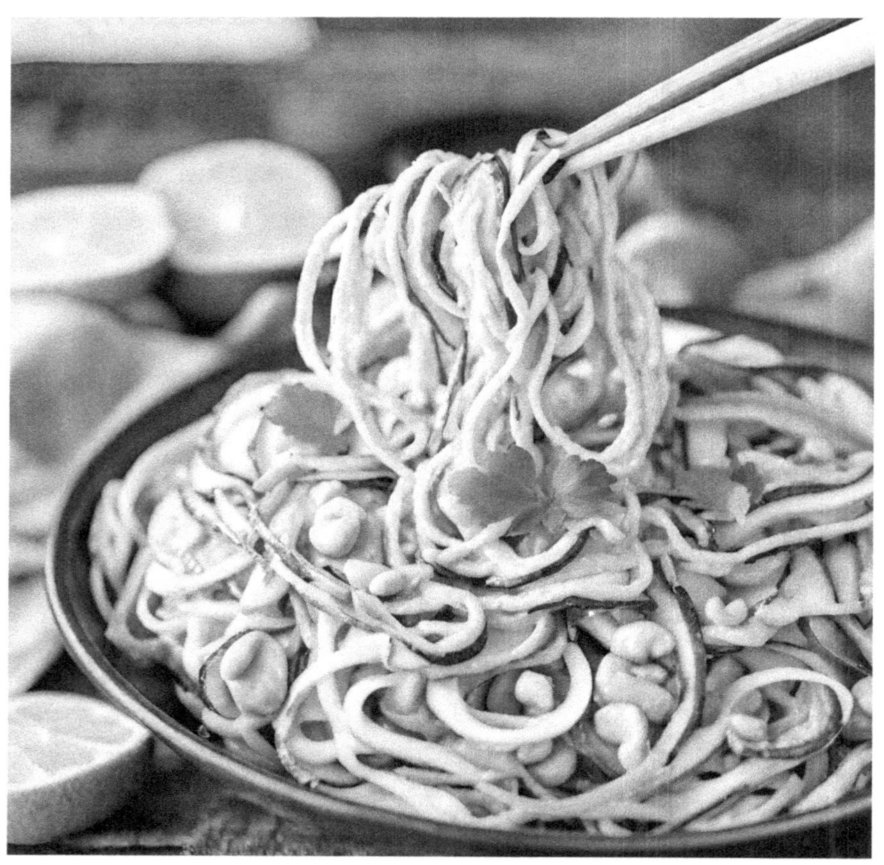

TABLE OF CONTENTS

Introduction..6

Chapter 1: What is Hashimoto's Disease?
    ○ Symptoms and Diagnosis..8
    ○ Hashimoto's and Your Immune System..............................10

Chapter 2: The Hashimoto's Diet Explained
    ○ Foods to Embrace and Avoid..13
    ○ The Role of Gluten, Dairy, and Soy....................................17

Breakfast Recipes
Gluten-Free Oatmeal...20
Buckwheat Pancakes...21
Sweet Potato Hash..22
Quinoa Porridge..23
Baked Eggs in Avocado...24
Sardine Salad...25
Turkey Bacon Wraps...26
Coconut Yogurt Parfait..27
Banana Almond Butter Smoothie...28
Pumpkin Seed Oatmeal...29
Zucchini and Sweet Potato Fritters..30
Paleo Breakfast Muffins..31
Hemp Seed Porridge...32
Spinach and Mushroom Omelette...33
Almond Flour Waffles..34
Green Detox Smoothie...35
Roasted Vegetable Hash..36
Berry Chia Overnight Oats...37
Egg Muffins..38
Salmon Avocado Salad..39
Paleo Banana Bread..40
Coconut Almond Porridge..41

Poultry & Meat Recipes
Ethiopian Doro Wat...42.
Irish Beef Stew...43
Vietnamese Shaking Beef (Bò Lúc Lắc)...44
Peruvian Roast Chicken..45
Lebanese Garlic Chicken...46
Hungarian Beef Goulash...47
Sicilian Chicken Soup..48
Thai Basil Chicken..49
Cuban Mojo Pork..50
Turkish Chicken Kebabs..51
Paleo Beef Stroganoff..52
Chicken Tikka Masala..53
Mediterranean Lamb Kebabs...54
Chicken Shawarma Salad..55
Beef Bulgogi..56
Jamaican Jerk Chicken...57
Italian Herb Chicken Thighs..58
Asian Turkey Lettuce Wraps..59
Chicken Cacciatore...60
Herb-Roasted Turkey Breast..61
Greek Lamb Meatballs...62
Indian Chicken Curry...63
Moroccan Lamb Tagine..64
Beef Stir-Fry..65

Fish & Seafood Recipes
Grilled Salmon with Avocado Salsa..66
Shrimp Zoodle Alfredo...67
Thai Coconut Curry Mussels..68
Moroccan Grilled Sardines..69
Baked Cod with Lemon and Dill...70
Paleo Paella..71
Italian Seafood Stew..72
Salmon Poke Bowl..73
Garlic-Lime Shrimp...74
Bouillabaisse...75
Tandoori Prawns...76
Smoked Salmon Breakfast Salad...77

Prawn Tikka...78
Lemon Dill Scallop Skewers.................................79
Halibut Piccata..80
Cajun Catfish..81
Greek Grilled Octopus......................................82
Brazilian Moqueca..83
Baked Lemon Sole with Capers...............................84
Crab Salad with Citrus Vinaigrette.........................85
Korean Grilled Mackerel....................................86

Vegetables and salads
Roasted Cauliflower Steak..................................87
Kale and Brussels Sprout Salad.............................88
Spicy Roasted Sweet Potatoes...............................89
Quinoa Tabbouleh...90
Balsamic Grilled Vegetables................................91
Asian Cucumber Salad.......................................92
Eggplant Caponata..93
Greek Salad..94
Mexican Street Corn Salad..................................95
Spinach and Strawberry Salad...............................96
Butternut Squash Risotto...................................97
Avocado Tomato Salad.......................................98
Zucchini Ribbon Salad......................................99
Warm Mushroom Salad..100
Broccoli and Apple Salad...................................101
Sweet Potato and Black Bean Salad..........................102
Mediterranean Lentil Salad.................................103
Cucumber Gazpacho..104
Roasted Brussels Sprouts with Pomegranate..................105
Thai Peanut Zucchini Noodles...............................106
Sautéed Green Beans with Garlic............................107
Watermelon and Feta Salad..................................108
Moroccan Carrot Salad......................................109

7-WEEK MEAL PLAN...110

BONUSES..116

To show our appreciation for your purchase, we're delighted to offer you these special bonuses as a heartfelt thank you.

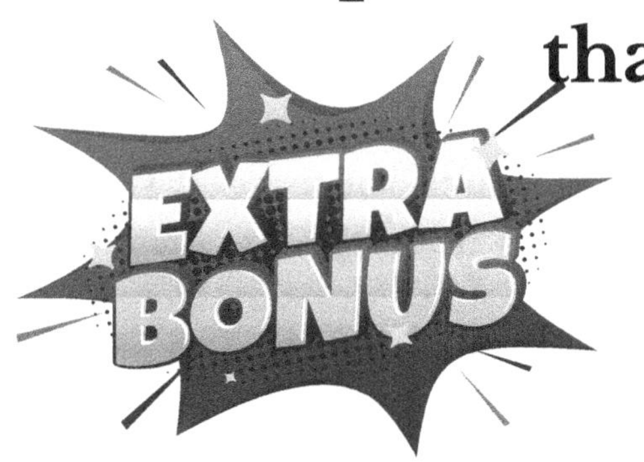

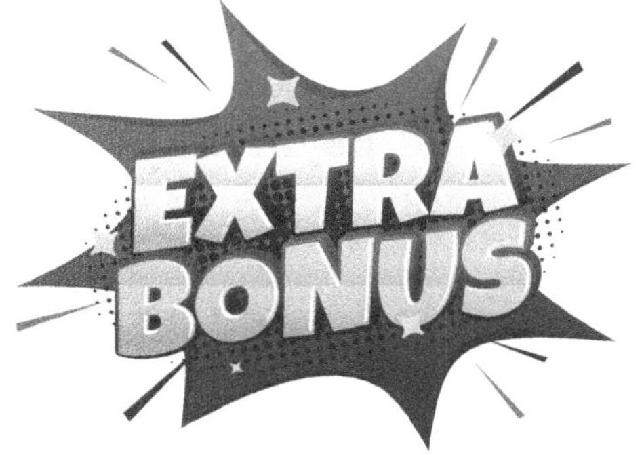

1. A Food Tracker Journal
2. Downloadable E-BOOK featuring full-color images of finished recipes
3. One-on-one consultation session with Dr. Kelly Haaland

Introduction

If you're picking up this book, you're likely familiar with the challenges and intricacies of living with Hashimoto's, an autoimmune condition that turns the body's defenses against its own thyroid gland. You're not alone in this journey, and this book aims to be a companion, guide, and inspiration in your kitchen and beyond. Hashimoto's thyroiditis affects countless individuals worldwide, presenting a variety of symptoms that can profoundly impact daily life. From fatigue and weight fluctuations to digestive issues and beyond, the condition requires a nuanced approach to health and wellness. One of the most impactful steps many have found in managing Hashimoto's is through dietary modifications, specifically, adopting a gluten-free diet. Why gluten-free, you might ask? The answer lies in the complex interplay between autoimmune conditions, inflammation, and the gut. Gluten, a protein found in wheat, barley, and rye, has been shown to potentially exacerbate symptoms for those with Hashimoto's by contributing to inflammation and increasing intestinal permeability, also known as "leaky gut."

This cookbook is more than simply a list of recipes; it's an ode to the therapeutic value of food and the significant impact nutrition can have on overall health. Each recipe has been carefully crafted to delight the taste buds while supporting your health journey. Whether you're an experienced cook or a beginner in the kitchen, you'll find dishes that cater to your skill level, dietary needs, and flavor preferences. From filling breakfasts and substantial dinners to delicious poultry, every page offers a gluten-free solution to satisfy your cravings without compromising your health. But "The **Hashimoto's Cookbook Gluten-Free** is more than just recipes. It's a source of education, empowerment, and encouragement. We dive into the whys and hows of a gluten-free diet for Hashimoto's, offering insights into how certain foods can support or hinder thyroid function. We explore the importance of whole, nutrient-dense foods and provide practical tips for navigating gluten-free living, from reading labels to avoiding cross-contamination.

We understand that a diagnosis of Hashimoto's can feel overwhelming, and the path to managing it is deeply personal. This book seeks to honor that individual journey, providing options and flexibility within recipes to cater to additional dietary restrictions and preferences. Food allergies, sensitivities, and personal tastes are all considered, ensuring that everyone can find something that not only nourishes but also delights. As you turn each page, we invite you to embrace the adventure that cooking can be. Experiment with new ingredients, try unfamiliar dishes, and rediscover the joy of eating in a way that loves you back. Food is a powerful tool in your Hashimoto's management arsenal, and with "The Hashimoto's Cookbook Gluten-Free you're well-equipped to wield it with confidence and creativity.

Welcome to your gluten-free journey with Hashimoto's. Let's get cooking and transform the way you eat, live, and thrive.

Dear Esteemed Reader

We understand that each individual's path to wellness is as unique as their fingerprint, especially when navigating dietary restrictions. With this in mind, we encourage you to view our recipes not as rigid guidelines but as flexible friends, ready to be adapted to meet your personal dietary needs and preferences. Your intuition and individual health considerations should be your compass as you explore the flavors and possibilities within these pages.

We also recommend maintaining an open line of communication with your healthcare provider. If ever in doubt or if specific dietary questions arise, your doctor or a qualified nutritionist can offer guidance tailored to your health journey, ensuring that your dietary choices support your well-being in the most effective way.

Please note that the nutritional information provided alongside our recipes is an approximation. Variations in ingredients and their sizes can lead to slight differences in nutritional content. We strive for accuracy, but we also celebrate the organic nature of cooking and the beauty of using what's fresh, available, and most nourishing to your body.

Thank you for allowing us to be a part of your journey. Here's to a path filled with discovery, wellness, and, most importantly, delectable meals that feed both body and soul.

Bon Appétit,

The Team Behind "Hashimoto's Cookbook Gluten-Free"

Chapter 1: What is Hashimoto's Disease?

Symptoms and Diagnosis

Hashimoto's disease, also known as Hashimoto's thyroiditis, is an autoimmune disorder where the immune system attacks the thyroid gland, leading to chronic thyroid damage and affecting hormone production. This can result in hypothyroidism, where the thyroid does not produce enough hormones, leading to various physical and mental symptoms. For successful management and therapy of Hashimoto's disease, it is essential to comprehend the symptoms and the diagnosis procedure.

Symptoms of Hashimoto's Disease
The symptoms of Hashimoto's can be broad, vary widely among individuals, and develop slowly over years. They are typically related to the reduced output of thyroid hormones (hypothyroidism) and may include:
- **Fatigue**: A pervasive sense of tiredness is common, which is not relieved by sleeping or rest.
- **Weight Gain:** Unexplained weight gain can occur, often despite no change in diet or exercise habits.
- Cold Intolerance: Feeling unusually cold is a frequent complaint, as thyroid hormones help regulate body temperature.
- **Dry Skin and Hair:** The skin may become dry, flaky, and rough, while hair can become coarse, brittle, or thin.
- Hair Loss: This can be significant and affect the entire scalp rather than localized areas.
- Constipation: Reduced thyroid hormone levels can slow down the digestive process.
- **Depression and Mood Changes:** Hypothyroidism can affect mental health, causing depression or mood swings.
- **Memory and Focus Issues:** People may experience forgetfulness, lack of focus, or general brain fog.

- **Menstrual Irregularities:** Women may experience heavier, more frequent, or more painful periods.
- **Muscle Weakness and Joint Pain:** Aches, pains, stiffness, and weakness in muscles and joints are common.
- **Swelling of the Thyroid Gland (Goiter):** The neck may appear swollen or enlarged due to an inflamed thyroid.

Diagnosis of Hashimoto's Disease

Diagnosing Hashimoto's involves several steps, often starting with a review of symptoms and medical history, followed by clinical evaluation and specific tests:

- **Medical History and Physical Exam:** A doctor will review the patient's symptoms, medical history, and perform a physical examination, paying particular attention to the thyroid gland's size and any signs of hormone imbalance.
- **Blood Tests:**
    - **Thyroid-Stimulating Hormone (TSH) Test:** Elevated levels of TSH can indicate the thyroid isn't producing enough hormones, prompting the pituitary gland to release more TSH.
    - **Thyroxine (T4) Levels:** Low levels of the thyroid hormone T4 suggest hypothyroidism.
    - **Thyroid Peroxidase Antibodies (TPO Antibodies):** The presence of these antibodies can confirm that Hashimoto's is the cause of the thyroid dysfunction, as these antibodies are an indicator of an autoimmune reaction against the thyroid gland.
- **Imaging Tests:** Although not always required, an ultrasound of the thyroid might be performed to check for an enlarged thyroid gland or other abnormalities like nodules.
- **Additional Assessments:** In some cases, further evaluations might be necessary to understand the extent of the disease or to rule out other conditions.

Hashimoto's and Your Immune System

Hashimoto's thyroiditis, an autoimmune disorder, is fundamentally an interplay between your immune system and thyroid gland, one that can have wide-reaching implications for overall health. This condition epitomizes how the immune system, when misdirected, can become the very source of physiological dysfunction, targeting the thyroid gland and significantly impacting its function. Investigating the mechanisms of the autoimmune response, the impact on the thyroid, and the wider health implications is necessary to comprehend the link between Hashimoto's and the immune system.

Autoimmune Response in Hashimoto's

Autoimmunity occurs when the immune system mistakenly identifies the body's own tissues as foreign invaders and attacks them. In Hashimoto's thyroiditis:

- **Antibody Production:** The immune system produces antibodies against thyroid peroxidase (TPO) and thyroglobulin, which are crucial in the production of thyroid hormones. These antibodies attack the cells in the thyroid gland, leading to inflammation and damage.
- **Chronic Inflammation:** The continuous assault on the thyroid results in chronic inflammation, which gradually destroys thyroid tissue. This process can lead to the gland's inability to produce sufficient thyroid hormones, resulting in hypothyroidism.

Impact on Thyroid Function

The thyroid gland plays a pivotal role in regulating metabolism, growth, and development through its hormones, thyroxine (T4) and triiodothyronine (T3). Hashimoto's typically leads to hypothyroidism, where the damaged thyroid can't produce enough hormones, affecting various body systems:

- **Metabolic Disruption:** Reduced levels of thyroid hormones can slow down metabolic processes, leading to symptoms like weight gain, fatigue, and cold intolerance.

- **Neurological Effects:** Thyroid hormones are crucial for brain function, and their deficiency can result in mood swings, cognitive impairment, and depression.
- **Cardiovascular Changes:** Hypothyroidism can lead to increased cholesterol levels and, over time, heighten the risk of heart disease.

Genetic and Environmental Factors

The exact cause of Hashimoto's is not fully understood, but it is believed to result from a combination of genetic predisposition and environmental triggers:

- **Genetic Susceptibility:** Individuals with a family history of Hashimoto's or other autoimmune diseases are at higher risk, suggesting a genetic component to the disease.
- **Environmental Triggers:** Various factors, including infections, stress, pregnancy, and certain medications, can trigger the autoimmune response in susceptible individuals. Dietary components, particularly iodine and selenium intake, can also influence thyroid function and autoimmune activity.

Broader Health Implications

The interplay between Hashimoto's and the immune system can have broader health implications, necessitating a comprehensive approach to management:

- **Other Autoimmune Disorders:** Individuals with Hashimoto's are at an increased risk of developing other autoimmune conditions, such as rheumatoid arthritis, type 1 diabetes, and celiac disease.
- **Impact on Quality of Life:** The symptoms of Hashimoto's, particularly fatigue and weight changes, can significantly affect an individual's quality of life and mental health.
- **Pregnancy Considerations:** Hashimoto's can impact fertility and pregnancy outcomes, making it important for affected women to closely monitor their thyroid hormone levels during pregnancy.

Management Strategies

Effective management of Hashimoto's involves a multifaceted approach focusing on restoring thyroid hormone levels, reducing antibody levels, and addressing the underlying immune dysfunction:

- **Hormone Replacement Therapy:** Levothyroxine is commonly prescribed to normalize thyroid hormone levels, alleviating many of the symptoms associated with hypothyroidism.
- **Lifestyle Modifications:** Diet, exercise, stress reduction, and avoiding environmental triggers can help manage symptoms and potentially reduce autoimmune activity.
- **Regular Monitoring:** Regular check-ups with healthcare providers, including monitoring of thyroid function tests and antibody levels, are crucial to tailor the treatment plan and adjust medication dosages.

Hence, Hashimoto's disease exemplifies a complex interrelation between the immune system and thyroid gland, leading to significant health implications. Understanding this relationship is key to managing the condition effectively, preventing long-term complications, and maintaining overall well-being. Individuals diagnosed with Hashimoto's require ongoing care and lifestyle adjustments to live well with the condition, emphasizing the importance of personalized treatment and comprehensive support.

Chapter 2: The Hashimoto's Diet Explained

Foods to Embrace and Avoid

When managing Hashimoto's thyroiditis, a strategic approach to diet can significantly influence the condition's management and the individual's overall well-being. The focus is often on embracing foods that support thyroid function and immune health while avoiding those that can potentially exacerbate symptoms or hinder thyroid function.

Foods to Embrace

1. Anti-Inflammatory Foods:
- **Benefits:** Help reduce the autoimmune response and decrease inflammation in the thyroid gland.
- **Include:** Leafy greens, berries, nuts, seeds, and fatty fish like salmon, which are rich in antioxidants and omega-3 fatty acids.

2. Selenium-Rich Foods:
- **Importance:** Selenium is crucial for the conversion of T4 to the active hormone T3 and for reducing thyroid antibody levels.
- **Sources:** Brazil nuts, seafood, turkey, and chicken are excellent sources of selenium.

3. High-Fiber Foods:
- **Role:** Support digestion, aid in maintaining healthy blood sugar levels, and promote satiety, which can be beneficial for weight management.
- **Options:** Vegetables, fruits, legumes, and whole grains (for those who can tolerate them).

4. Zinc-Containing Foods:
- **Significance:** Zinc is essential for thyroid hormone synthesis and immune system function.
- **Rich Foods:** Beef, shellfish, chickpeas, and pumpkin seeds are good sources of zinc.

5. Iron-Rich Foods:
- **Necessity:** Iron is vital for thyroid hormone production and energy metabolism.
- **Sources:** Lean meats, seafood, beans, spinach, and quinoa are beneficial for maintaining adequate iron levels.

6. Foods Rich in Antioxidants:

- **Purpose:** Combat oxidative stress and support overall cellular health.
- **Examples:** Berries, apples, carrots, and beets are loaded with vitamins and antioxidants.

7. Healthy Fats:

- **Benefits:** Essential for hormone balance and reducing inflammation.
- **Sources:** Avocados, olive oil, coconut oil, and omega-3s from fish or flaxseeds.

8. Hydrating Fluids:

- **Importance:** Adequate hydration supports all bodily functions, including the thyroid.
- **Recommendations:** Water, herbal teas, and nutrient-rich broths.

Foods to Avoid

1. Gluten-Containing Foods:

- **Reason:** Many individuals with Hashimoto's find their symptoms improve on a gluten-free diet, potentially due to gluten's role in gut inflammation and autoimmunity.
- **Avoid:** Wheat, barley, rye, and products containing these grains.

2. Dairy Products:

- **Context:** Some people with Hashimoto's are sensitive to dairy, which can trigger inflammation or immune responses.
- **Alternatives:** Consider lactose-free options or plant-based substitutes.

3. Goitrogens:

- **Explanation:** Certain compounds that can interfere with thyroid function, though they're mostly a concern when consumed in large amounts and raw.
- **Common Sources:** Raw cruciferous vegetables like broccoli, cauliflower, and kale; cooking these vegetables can reduce their goitrogenic effect.

4. Highly Processed Foods:

- **Impact:** Can exacerbate inflammation, contribute to weight gain, and affect overall health.
- **Typical Examples:** Fast foods, fried foods, sugary snacks, and beverages.

5. **Excess Iodine:**
- **Balance:** While iodine is critical for thyroid hormone production, too much can exacerbate Hashimoto's symptoms.
- **Caution:** Be wary of supplements or iodine-rich foods in high quantities, such as seaweed or iodized salt.

6. **Soy Products:**
- **Consideration:** Soy can interfere with the absorption of thyroid medication and may affect thyroid function.
- **Limit:** Soybeans, tofu, soy milk, and other soy-based foods, especially close to taking thyroid medication.

7. **Excessive Sugars and Refined Carbohydrates:**
- **Concerns:** Can lead to spikes in blood sugar, contribute to weight gain, and increase inflammation.
- **Avoid:** Sugary desserts, candies, sodas, and refined grains like white bread.

8. **Alcohol:**
- **Effects:** Can contribute to liver stress, hormonal imbalances, and immune dysfunction.
- **Moderation:** Limit or avoid alcohol to support overall health and thyroid function.

Implementing Dietary Changes

- **Personalization:** Diet modifications should be personalized, as individual tolerance can vary widely. Monitoring how different foods affect your symptoms is key.
- **Consultation:** It's wise to consult with a healthcare provider or a dietitian specialized in thyroid health to create a balanced diet plan that meets your nutritional needs, supports your thyroid health, and aligns with your personal health goals.
- **Gradual Changes:** Implementing dietary changes gradually can help in identifying how specific foods impact your symptoms and overall well-being.
- **Keeping a Food Diary:** Logging your daily food intake, symptoms, and how you feel can be an invaluable tool in identifying patterns and foods that may exacerbate your condition.
- **Whole Foods Focus:** Emphasizing whole, unprocessed foods can help ensure you're getting a wide range of nutrients necessary for optimal thyroid function and overall health.

- **Cooking Methods:** Being mindful of cooking methods can also be beneficial. For example, steaming or boiling cruciferous vegetables can reduce their goitrogenic properties.
- **Mindful Eating:** Paying attention to your body's hunger signals and eating mindfully can support better digestion and absorption of nutrients, which is beneficial for overall health and particularly important for those with thyroid conditions.
- **Supplement Wisely:** Some individuals with Hashimoto's may benefit from supplementation, such as selenium, zinc, or vitamin D, especially if they are deficient in these nutrients. However, it's essential to consult with a healthcare professional before starting any supplements, as they can interact with other medications or exacerbate certain conditions.
- **Avoiding Fad Diets:** Extreme diets or quick-fix solutions can often do more harm than good, especially for those with an autoimmune condition. It's important to adopt a balanced, sustainable eating pattern that includes a variety of nutrients.
- **Consideration of Food Sensitivities:** Apart from common triggers like gluten and dairy, individuals with Hashimoto's may have other food sensitivities. An elimination diet, conducted under the supervision of a healthcare provider, can help identify these sensitivities.
- **Balanced Nutrient Intake:** Ensuring that your diet is not only restrictive but also nutritionally balanced is crucial. It should provide all the essential macronutrients (proteins, fats, carbohydrates) and micronutrients (vitamins and minerals) your body needs.
- **Hydration:** Maintaining adequate hydration is important for overall health and can support the body's detoxification processes, digestion, and even hormone production.

The Role of Gluten, Dairy, and Soy

In the context of Hashimoto's thyroiditis, the role of dietary components, particularly gluten, dairy, and soy, is of considerable interest and debate. Many individuals with Hashimoto's observe significant improvements in their symptoms and overall thyroid function when they adjust their intake of these foods.

Gluten and Hashimoto's Thyroiditis
Immune System Response:
- Gluten, a protein found in wheat, barley, and rye, can provoke an inflammatory response in susceptible individuals, particularly those with celiac disease or non-celiac gluten sensitivity.
- In some cases, the molecular structure of gluten can mimic that of thyroid tissue, leading to a phenomenon known as molecular mimicry. This can cause the immune system to mistakenly attack the thyroid gland, exacerbating Hashimoto's thyroiditis.

Intestinal Permeability:
- Gluten consumption can contribute to increased intestinal permeability, often referred to as "leaky gut," which allows particles, including undigested food, bacteria, and toxins, to pass into the bloodstream, potentially leading to an enhanced autoimmune response.

Recommendations:
- Many healthcare practitioners suggest a trial of gluten-free diet to see if symptoms improve, as this can reduce inflammation, decrease autoantibody levels, and potentially improve thyroid function.

Dairy and Hashimoto's Thyroiditis
Lactose and Casein Sensitivity:
- Dairy products contain lactose and casein, which some individuals with Hashimoto's may find difficult to digest, leading to inflammation, gastrointestinal distress, and an exacerbated autoimmune response.

Autoimmune Response:
- Similar to gluten, casein in dairy products might trigger an immune response in sensitive individuals, potentially worsening Hashimoto's symptoms or contributing to the autoimmune attack on the thyroid gland.

Calcium and Vitamin D:
- While dairy is a good source of calcium and vitamin D, essential for bone health, individuals who decide to eliminate dairy should find alternative sources of these nutrients to maintain bone strength and overall health.

Recommendations:
- A dairy-free trial period might help determine if dairy exacerbates Hashimoto's symptoms. Monitoring changes in symptoms can provide insights into whether dairy should be avoided long-term.

Soy and Hashimoto's Thyroiditis

Effects on Thyroid Function:
- Soy contains isoflavones, compounds that may have goitrogenic effects, meaning they could interfere with thyroid hormone production and absorption. Isoflavones can inhibit the enzyme thyroid peroxidase, which is involved in the synthesis of thyroid hormones.

Interference with Thyroid Medication:
- Soy products can interfere with the absorption of thyroid hormone replacement medications. Patients are often advised to consume soy products at different times from their medication to ensure proper absorption.

Phytoestrogen Activity:
- Soy isoflavones are phytoestrogens, plant-derived compounds that can mimic estrogen in the body. While their impact is much weaker than human estrogen, excessive consumption in sensitive individuals could theoretically disrupt endocrine function, including thyroid hormone activity.

Recommendations:
- Moderation is key with soy consumption, and individuals with Hashimoto's are often advised to monitor their response to soy. It may not be necessary to eliminate soy entirely, but being mindful of its potential effects is important, especially regarding thyroid medication timing and overall consumption.

Personalized Dietary Approach

The impact of gluten, dairy, and soy can vary significantly from person to person with Hashimoto's. While some may experience notable improvements in their symptoms and thyroid function when avoiding these foods, others may not notice a difference. Implementing dietary changes should ideally be a personalized process, guided by careful observation of symptoms, and, when possible, the support of healthcare professionals knowledgeable about Hashimoto's and nutrition.

A thoughtful approach to diet, focusing on individual responses and potential sensitivities, can be a key component in managing Hashimoto's thyroiditis effectively. It's about finding the right balance that supports the immune system, reduces inflammation, and maintains overall health while ensuring that the diet remains nutritionally adequate and sustainable in the long term.

Breakfast Recipes

1. Gluten-Free Oatmeal

Ingredients:

- 1 cup gluten-free rolled oats
- 2 cups water or dairy-free milk
- 1/4 tsp salt
- 1 tbsp maple syrup or honey (optional)
- Fresh fruits, nuts, and seeds for topping

Instructions:

1. Combine the oats, water/milk, and salt in a saucepan.
2. Bring to a boil, then reduce heat to low and simmer, stirring occasionally, until the oats are soft, about 10-15 minutes.
3. Remove from heat and stir in the maple syrup or honey if using.
4. Serve hot with your choice of fruits, nuts, and seeds.

Nutritional Info (per serving):

- Calories: ~150-200 (without toppings)
- Protein: 5g
- Fat: 3g
- Carbohydrates: 27g
- Fiber: 4g

Serves: 2

Cooking Time: 15 minutes

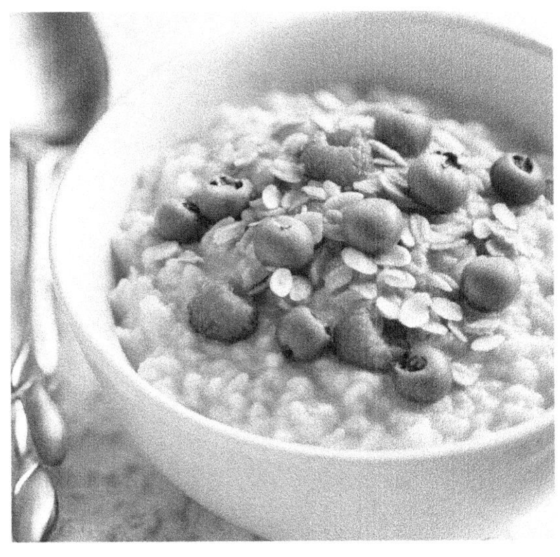

2. Buckwheat Pancakes

Ingredients:

- 1 cup buckwheat flour
- 1 tbsp baking powder
- 1/4 tsp salt
- 1 cup dairy-free milk
- 1 egg (or flaxseed egg for vegan option)
- 2 tbsp melted coconut oil
- 1 tbsp honey or maple syrup

Instructions:

1. Mix the buckwheat flour, baking powder, and salt in a bowl.
2. In another bowl, whisk together the milk, egg, coconut oil, and sweetener.
3. Combine wet and dry ingredients and stir until just mixed.
4. Heat a non-stick skillet over medium heat and pour 1/4 cup batter for each pancake.
5. Cook until bubbles form, then flip and cook until golden brown.
6. Serve hot with your favorite toppings.

Nutritional Info (per serving):

- Calories: ~220
- Protein: 6g
- Fat: 9g
- Carbohydrates: 31g
- Fiber: 5g

Serves: 4

Cooking Time: 20 minutes

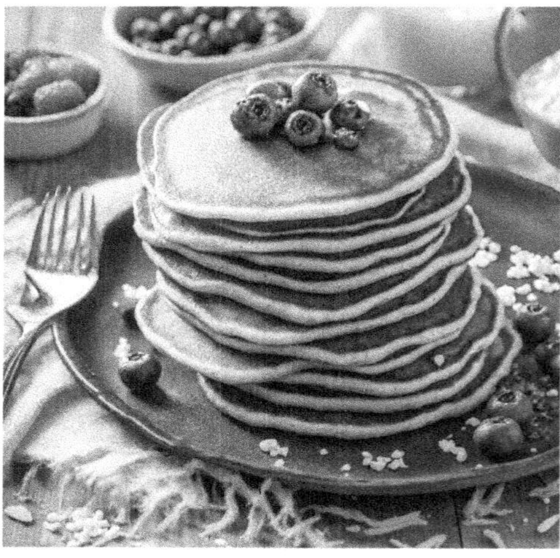

3. Sweet Potato Hash

Ingredients:
- 2 medium sweet potatoes, peeled and diced
- 1 red bell pepper, diced
- 1 onion, diced
- 2 cloves garlic, minced
- 2 tbsp olive oil
- Salt and pepper to taste
- Fresh herbs (like parsley or thyme)

Instructions:
1. Heat olive oil in a large skillet over medium heat.
2. Add sweet potatoes, stirring occasionally, until they start to soften, about 10 minutes.
3. Add onion, bell pepper, and garlic, cooking until all vegetables are tender, about 5-8 minutes.
4. Season with salt, pepper, and fresh herbs.
5. Serve warm.

Nutritional Info (per serving):
- Calories: ~200
- Protein: 3g
- Fat: 7g
- Carbohydrates: 33g
- Fiber: 5g

Serves: 4
Cooking Time: 20 minutes

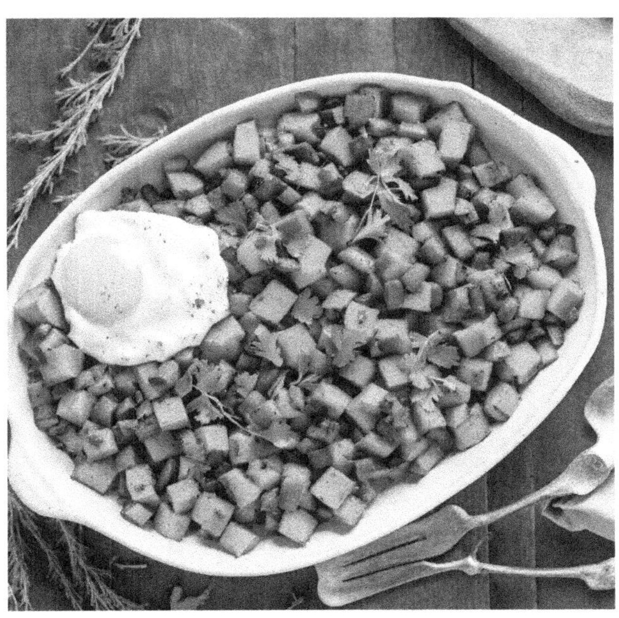

4. Quinoa Porridge

Ingredients:

- 1 cup quinoa, rinsed
- 2 cups dairy-free milk
- 1 cinnamon stick or 1/2 tsp ground cinnamon
- 2 tbsp maple syrup or honey
- Fresh fruits and nuts for topping

Instructions:

1. Combine quinoa, milk, and cinnamon in a saucepan and bring to a boil.
2. Reduce heat to low, cover, and simmer for 15-20 minutes or until quinoa is tender and creamy.
3. Remove from heat and remove the cinnamon stick if used.
4. Stir in maple syrup or honey.
5. Serve warm topped with fruits and nuts.

Nutritional Info (per serving):

- Calories: ~250
- Protein: 8g
- Fat: 5g
- Carbohydrates: 45g
- Fiber: 5g

Serves: 2
Cooking Time: 25 minutes

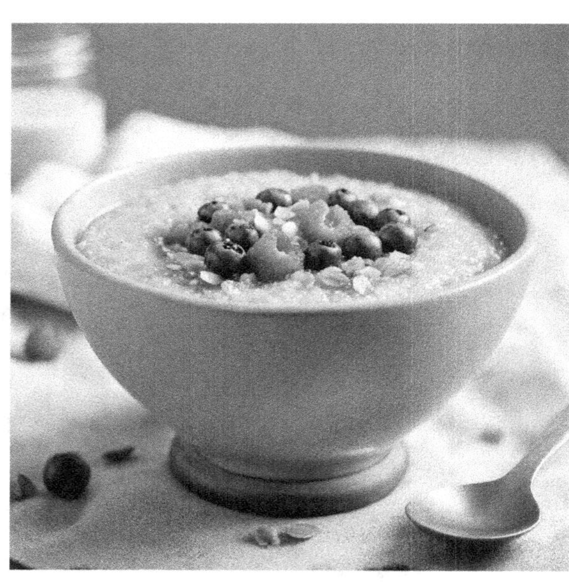

5. Baked Eggs in Avocado

Ingredients:

- 2 ripe avocados
- 4 small eggs
- Salt and pepper, to taste
- Chopped chives or parsley for garnish

Instructions:

1. Preheat the oven to 425°F (220°C).
2. Slice the avocados in half and remove the pit. Scoop out a bit more avocado to create enough space for the eggs.
3. Place the avocado halves in a baking dish and crack an egg into each half. Season with salt and pepper.
4. Bake for 15-20 minutes or until the egg whites are set.
5. Garnish with chives or parsley before serving.

Nutritional Info (per serving):

- Calories: ~300
- Protein: 14g
- Fat: 25g
- Carbohydrates: 13g
- Fiber: 10g

Serves: 4

Cooking Time: 20-25 minutes

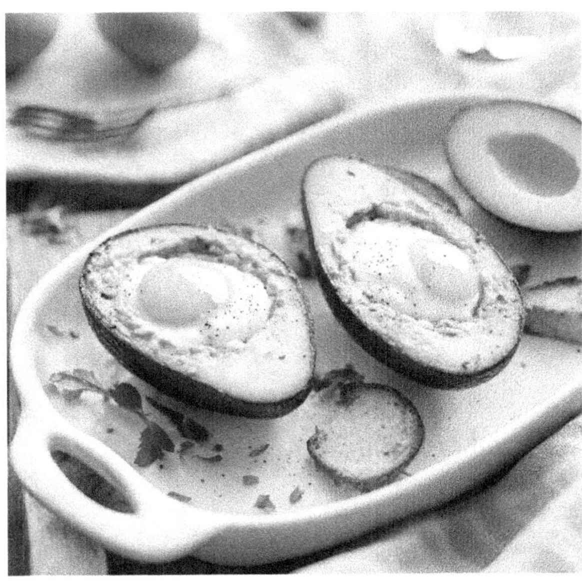

6. Sardine Salad

Ingredients:

- 2 cans of sardines in olive oil, drained
- 1 cup cherry tomatoes, halved
- 1 small red onion, finely sliced
- 1 cucumber, sliced
- 2 tablespoons lemon juice
- 2 tablespoons olive oil
- Salt and pepper to taste
- Mixed greens for serving

Instructions:

1. In a large bowl, combine sardines, cherry tomatoes, red onion, and cucumber.
2. Drizzle with lemon juice and olive oil, then season with salt and pepper. Toss gently to combine.
3. Serve over a bed of mixed greens.

Nutritional Info (per serving):

- Calories: ~250
- Protein: 20g
- Fat: 15g
- Carbohydrates: 6g
- Fiber: 2g

Serves: 4
Cooking Time: 10 minutes

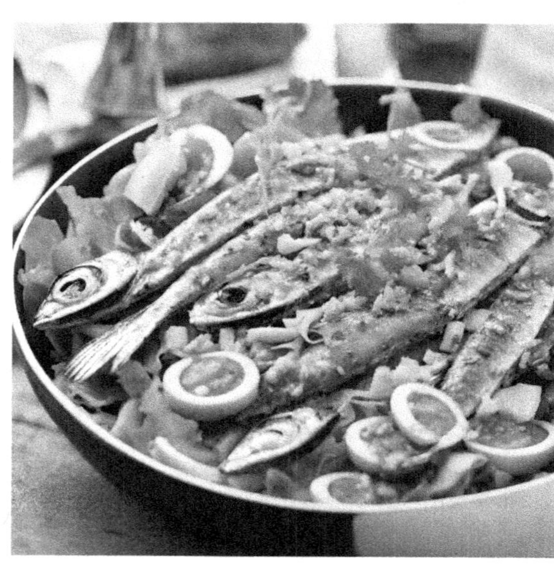

7. Turkey Bacon Wraps

Ingredients:
- 8 slices of turkey bacon
- 4 large lettuce leaves
- 1 avocado, sliced
- 1 tomato, sliced
- 1/4 cup mayonnaise or avocado mayo
- Salt and pepper to taste

Instructions:
1. Cook turkey bacon according to package instructions until crispy.
2. Lay out lettuce leaves and spread each with mayonnaise.
3. Place two slices of turkey bacon on each lettuce leaf, topped with avocado and tomato slices.
4. Season with salt and pepper, then roll up the lettuce to form wraps.

Nutritional Info (per serving):
- Calories: ~300
- Protein: 20g
- Fat: 22g
- Carbohydrates: 8g
- Fiber: 5g

Serves: 4
Cooking Time: 10-15 minutes

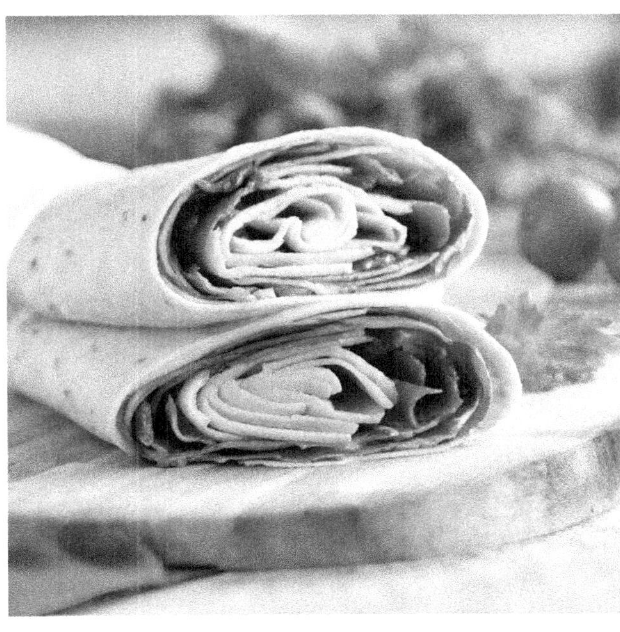

8. Coconut Yogurt Parfait

Ingredients:

- 2 cups unsweetened coconut yogurt
- 1 cup mixed berries (strawberries, blueberries, raspberries)
- 1/4 cup granola (gluten-free)
- 1 tablespoon honey or maple syrup (optional)
- A pinch of cinnamon

Instructions:

1. In serving glasses, layer coconut yogurt, mixed berries, and granola.
2. Repeat the layers until all ingredients are used up.
3. Drizzle with honey or maple syrup and sprinkle a pinch of cinnamon on top.

Nutritional Info (per serving):

- Calories: ~250
- Protein: 4g
- Fat: 15g
- Carbohydrates: 25g
- Fiber: 3g

Serves: 4

Cooking Time: 5 minutes

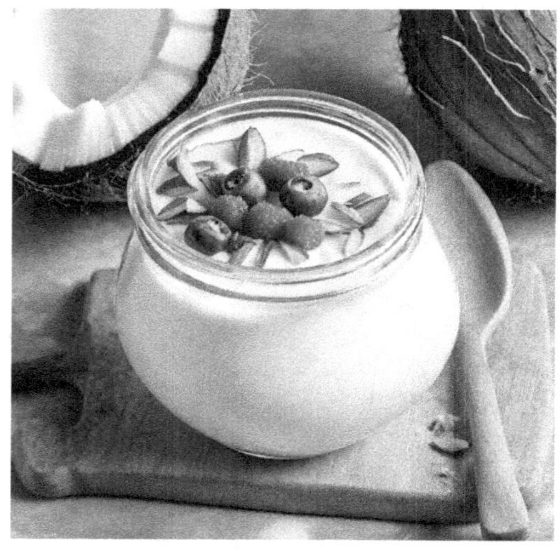

9. Banana Almond Butter Smoothie

Ingredients:

- 2 ripe bananas
- 2 tablespoons almond butter
- 1 cup unsweetened almond milk
- 1/2 teaspoon vanilla extract
- Ice cubes (optional)

Instructions:

1. Combine bananas, almond butter, almond milk, and vanilla extract in a blender.
2. Add ice cubes if desired and blend until smooth and creamy.

Nutritional Info (per serving):

- Calories: ~300
- Protein: 6g
- Fat: 15g
- Carbohydrates: 40g
- Fiber: 6g

Serves: 2

Cooking Time: 5 minutes

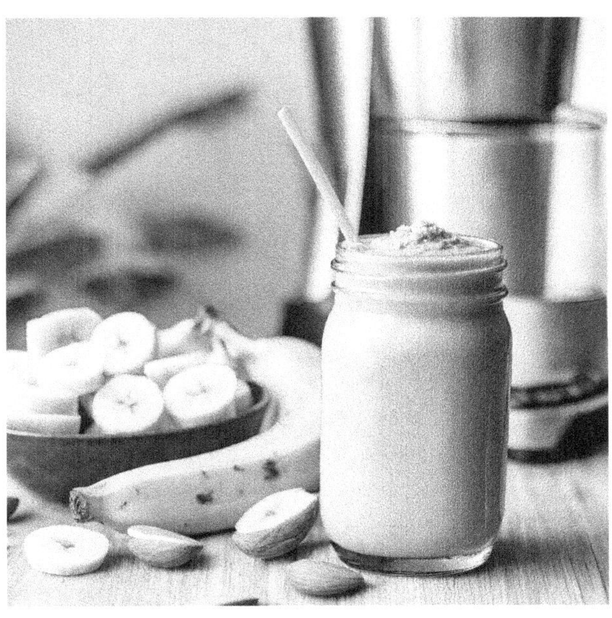

10. Pumpkin Seed Oatmeal

Ingredients:

- 1 cup gluten-free rolled oats
- 2 cups water or almond milk
- 1/2 cup pumpkin seeds
- 1 teaspoon cinnamon
- 1 apple, diced
- 2 tablespoons maple syrup or honey

Instructions:

1. In a saucepan, combine the oats and water or almond milk. Bring to a simmer over medium heat, stirring frequently.
2. Cook for about 5-10 minutes, or until the oats have absorbed the liquid and are fully cooked.
3. Stir in the cinnamon, diced apple, and pumpkin seeds. Cook for an additional 2 minutes.
4. Remove from heat and sweeten with maple syrup or honey.

Nutritional Info (per serving):

- Calories: ~320
- Protein: 10g
- Fat: 12g
- Carbohydrates: 44g
- Fiber: 8g

Serves: 2

Cooking Time: 15 minutes

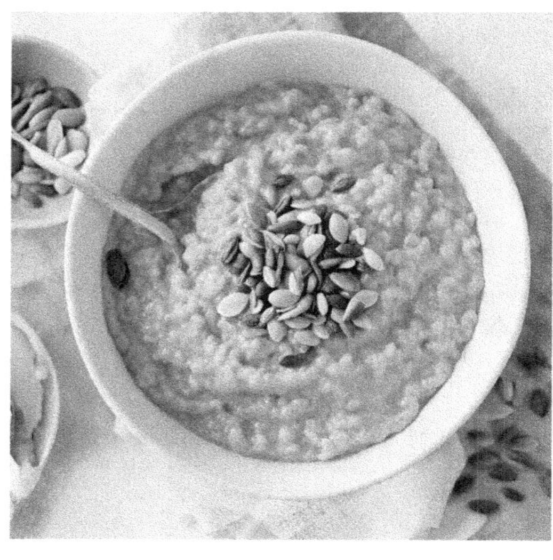

11. Zucchini and Sweet Potato Fritters

Ingredients:

- 1 large zucchini, grated
- 1 large sweet potato, peeled and grated
- 2 green onions, finely chopped
- 1/4 cup almond flour
- 2 eggs, beaten
- Salt and pepper to taste
- 2 tablespoons olive oil for frying

Instructions:

1. Combine grated zucchini and sweet potato in a bowl. Squeeze out excess moisture using a clean towel.
2. Add green onions, almond flour, and beaten eggs to the bowl. Season with salt and pepper and mix well.
3. Heat olive oil in a large skillet over medium heat. Scoop spoonfuls of the mixture into the skillet, flattening to form fritters.
4. Fry until golden brown on both sides, about 3-4 minutes per side.
5. Transfer to a paper towel-lined plate to drain any excess oil.

Nutritional Info (per serving):

- Calories: ~200
- Protein: 6g
- Fat: 12g
- Carbohydrates: 18g
- Fiber: 3g

Serves: 4

Cooking Time: 20 minutes

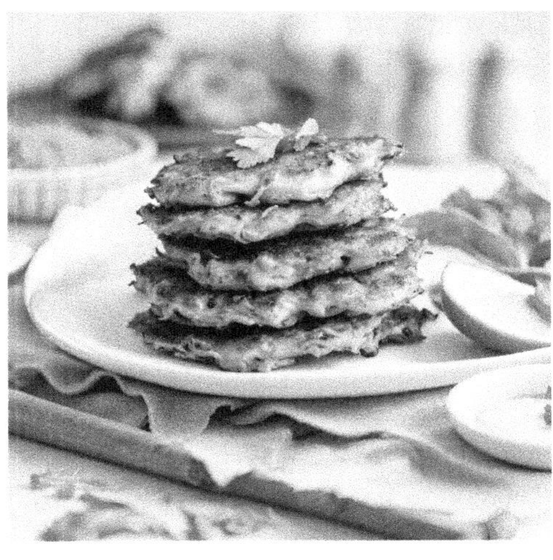

12. Paleo Breakfast Muffins

Ingredients:

- 6 eggs
- 1/4 cup coconut oil, melted
- 1/2 cup coconut flour
- 1/2 teaspoon baking soda
- 1/4 teaspoon salt
- 1 cup mixed vegetables (e.g., spinach, bell peppers, onions), finely diced
- 1/2 cup cooked diced ham or bacon (optional)

Instructions:

1. Preheat the oven to 350°F (175°C) and line a muffin tin with paper liners or grease with coconut oil.
2. In a large bowl, whisk the eggs and melted coconut oil together. Add the coconut flour, baking soda, and salt, mixing until well combined.
3. Fold in the mixed vegetables and cooked ham or bacon, if using.
4. Spoon the batter into the prepared muffin tin, filling each cup about two-thirds full.
5. Bake for 20-25 minutes, or until the muffins are firm to the touch and a toothpick inserted into the center comes out clean.

Nutritional Info (per serving):

- Calories: ~150 (without ham or bacon)
- Protein: 6g
- Fat: 10g
- Carbohydrates: 8g
- Fiber: 3g

Serves: 12 muffins

Cooking Time: 30 minutes

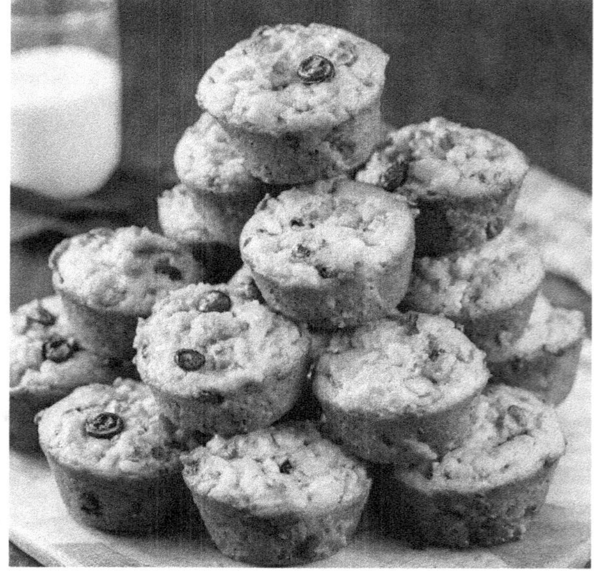

13. Hemp Seed Porridge

Ingredients:
- 1/2 cup hemp seeds
- 1 cup almond milk
- 1 tablespoon chia seeds
- 1 tablespoon flaxseed meal
- 1/2 teaspoon cinnamon
- 1 tablespoon maple syrup or honey (optional)
- Fresh berries and nuts for topping

Instructions:
1. In a small pot, combine hemp seeds, almond milk, chia seeds, flaxseed meal, and cinnamon.
2. Cook over medium heat, stirring frequently until the mixture thickens, about 5-7 minutes.
3. Remove from heat and stir in maple syrup or honey if using.
4. Serve hot, topped with fresh berries and nuts.

Nutritional Info (per serving):
- Calories: ~350
- Protein: 15g
- Fat: 25g
- Carbohydrates: 15g
- Fiber: 10g

Serves: 2

Cooking Time: 10 minutes

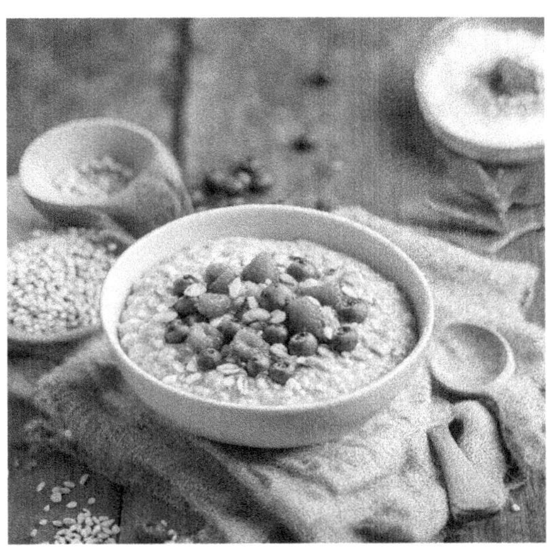

14. Spinach and Mushroom Omelette

Ingredients:

- 4 large eggs
- 1 cup spinach, chopped
- 1/2 cup mushrooms, sliced
- 1/4 cup onions, diced
- 1 tablespoon olive oil
- Salt and pepper to taste
- Fresh herbs (optional)

Instructions:

1. Beat the eggs in a bowl and season with salt and pepper.
2. Heat olive oil in a skillet over medium heat. Sauté onions and mushrooms until soft.
3. Add spinach and cook until wilted.
4. Pour the eggs over the vegetables, cover, and cook until the eggs are set.
5. Fold the omelette in half and serve hot, garnished with fresh herbs if desired.

Nutritional Info (per serving):

- Calories: ~300
- Protein: 20g
- Fat: 22g
- Carbohydrates: 5g
- Fiber: 1g

Serves: 2

Cooking Time: 15 minutes

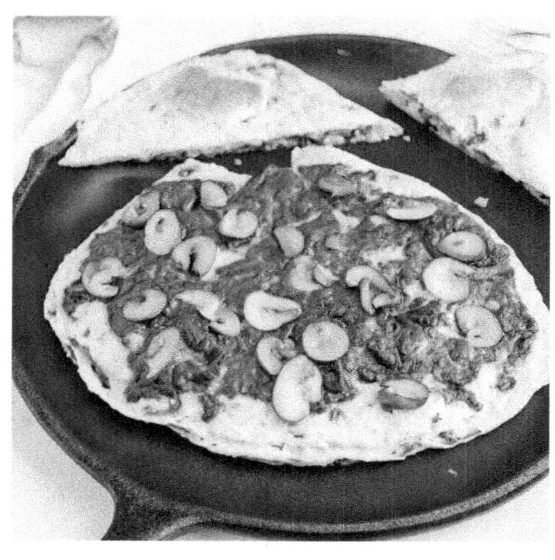

15. Almond Flour Waffles

Ingredients:

- 1 1/2 cups almond flour
- 1/2 teaspoon baking soda
- 1/4 teaspoon salt
- 2 large eggs
- 1/4 cup almond milk
- 2 tablespoons coconut oil, melted
- 1 tablespoon maple syrup
- 1 teaspoon vanilla extract

Instructions:

1. Preheat your waffle iron according to the manufacturer's instructions.
2. In a bowl, combine almond flour, baking soda, and salt.
3. In another bowl, whisk together eggs, almond milk, melted coconut oil, maple syrup, and vanilla extract.
4. Mix the wet ingredients into the dry ingredients until a batter is formed.
5. Cook in the waffle iron until golden brown and crispy.
6. Serve hot with your favorite toppings.

Nutritional Info (per serving):

- Calories: ~325
- Protein: 12g
- Fat: 28g
- Carbohydrates: 12g
- Fiber: 6g

Serves: 4

Cooking Time: 20 minutes

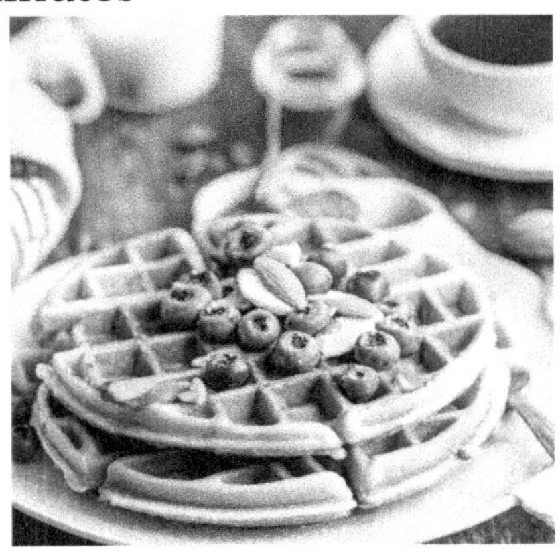

16. Green Detox Smoothie

Ingredients:

- 1 cup fresh spinach
- 1/2 cucumber, chopped
- 1/2 green apple, chopped
- 1/2 avocado
- 1 tablespoon chia seeds
- 1 cup coconut water or almond milk
- Juice of 1/2 lemon
- A few mint leaves (optional)

Instructions:

1. Combine all ingredients in a blender.
2. Blend until smooth.
3. Serve immediately, garnished with mint leaves if using.

Nutritional Info (per serving):

- Calories: ~250
- Protein: 5g
- Fat: 15g
- Carbohydrates: 27g
- Fiber: 10g

Serves: 2

Cooking Time: 5 minutes

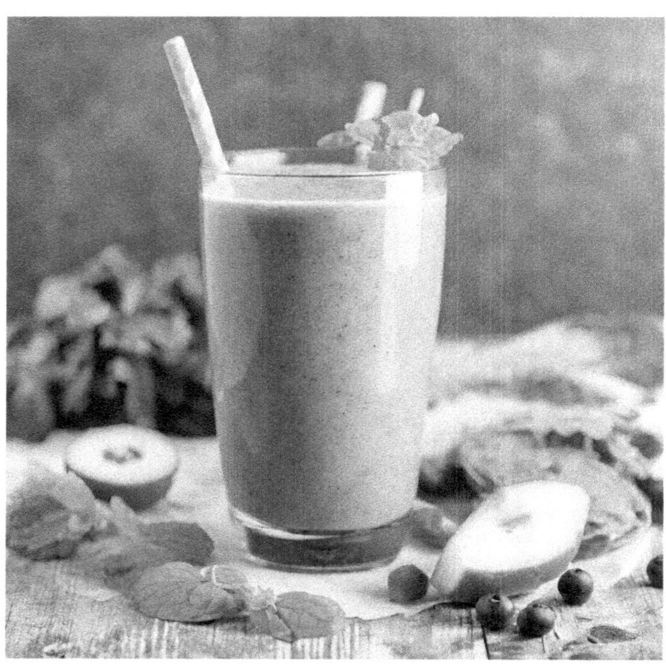

17. Roasted Vegetable Hash

Ingredients:

- 2 sweet potatoes, cubed
- 1 bell pepper, diced
- 1 zucchini, diced
- 1 red onion, diced
- 2 tablespoons olive oil
- Salt and pepper to taste
- Fresh herbs (thyme, rosemary)

Instructions:

1. Preheat the oven to 400°F (200°C).
2. Toss the vegetables with olive oil, salt, pepper, and herbs.
3. Spread the vegetables on a baking sheet and roast for 25-30 minutes, stirring halfway through, until tender and caramelized.

Nutritional Info (per serving):

- Calories: ~200
- Protein: 3g
- Fat: 7
- Carbohydrates: 33g
- Fiber: 6g

Serves: 4

Cooking Time: 30 minutes

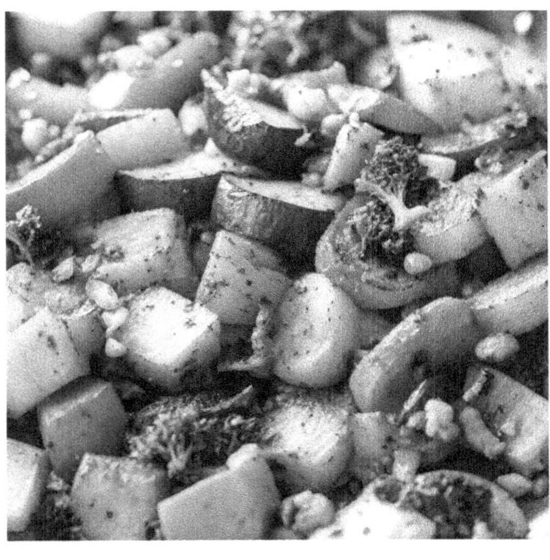

18. Berry Chia Overnight Oats

Ingredients:

- 1 cup rolled oats (gluten-free)
- 2 tablespoons chia seeds
- 1 cup almond milk
- 1/2 cup mixed berries (fresh or frozen)
- 1 tablespoon maple syrup or honey (optional)
- 1/2 teaspoon vanilla extract

Instructions:

1. In a jar or bowl, mix the oats, chia seeds, almond milk, berries, maple syrup (if using), and vanilla extract.
2. Stir well to combine, then cover and refrigerate overnight.
3. In the morning, stir the oats again and add extra almond milk if it's too thick. Serve cold or warmed up, with additional berries on top if desired.

Nutritional Info (per serving):

- Calories: ~300
- Protein: 8g
- Fat: 8g
- Carbohydrates: 48g
- Fiber: 10g

Serves: 2

Cooking Time: Overnight (plus a few minutes to prepare)

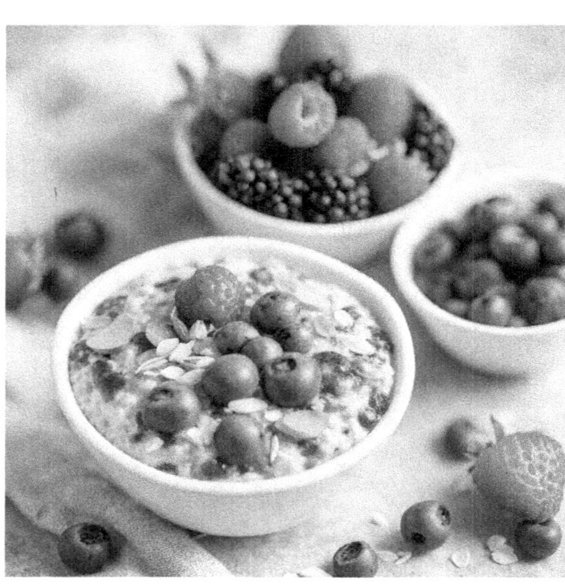

19. Egg Muffins

Ingredients:

- 6 large eggs
- 1/2 cup diced vegetables (bell peppers, spinach, onions)
- 1/4 cup shredded cheese (optional)
- Salt and pepper to taste
- Cooking spray or oil for greasing

Instructions:

1. Preheat the oven to 350°F (175°C). Grease a muffin tin with cooking spray or oil.
2. In a bowl, whisk the eggs and add the diced vegetables, cheese (if using), salt, and pepper.
3. Pour the egg mixture into the muffin cups, filling each about 2/3 full.
4. Bake for 20-25 minutes, or until the muffins are set and lightly golden on top.
5. Let them cool slightly before removing from the tin. Serve warm.

Nutritional Info (per serving):

- Calories: ~100 (without cheese)
- Protein: 7g
- Fat: 7g
- Carbohydrates: 2g
- Fiber: 0.5g

Serves: 6

Cooking Time: 30 minutes

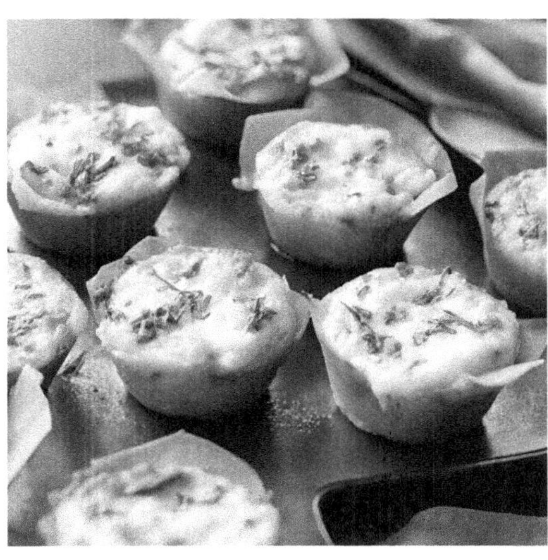

20. Salmon Avocado Salad

Ingredients:

- 2 cooked salmon fillets, flaked
- 1 ripe avocado, diced
- 1/2 cucumber, diced
- 1/4 red onion, thinly sliced
- 2 tablespoons lemon juice
- 2 tablespoons olive oil
- Salt and pepper to taste
- Mixed greens for serving

Instructions:

1. In a large bowl, combine the flaked salmon, diced avocado, cucumber, and red onion.
2. Drizzle with lemon juice and olive oil. Season with salt and pepper to taste.
3. Gently toss to combine. Serve over a bed of mixed greens.

Nutritional Info (per serving):

- Calories: ~400
- Protein: 25g
- Fat: 30g
- Carbohydrates: 9g
- Fiber: 7g

Serves: 2

Cooking Time: 10 minutes (assuming pre-cooked salmon)

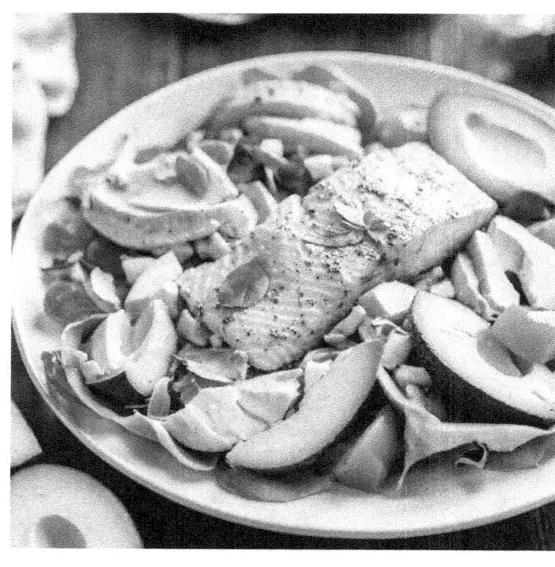

21. Paleo Banana Bread

Ingredients:

- 3 ripe bananas, mashed
- 3 eggs
- 1 tablespoon vanilla extract
- 1 cup almond flour
- 1/2 cup coconut flour
- 1 teaspoon baking soda
- 1/2 teaspoon salt
- 1/2 teaspoon cinnamon
- 1/4 cup melted coconut oil
- 1/2 cup walnuts, chopped (optional)

Instructions:

1. Preheat the oven to 350°F (175°C) and line a loaf pan with parchment paper.
2. In a large bowl, mix together the mashed bananas, eggs, vanilla, and coconut oil.
3. In another bowl, combine the almond flour, coconut flour, baking soda, salt, and cinnamon.
4. Mix the dry ingredients into the wet ingredients until well combined. Fold in the walnuts if using.
5. Pour the batter into the prepared loaf pan and bake for 50-60 minutes, or until a toothpick inserted into the center comes out clean.
6. Let the bread cool before slicing.

Nutritional Info (per serving):

- Calories: ~330
- Protein: 8g
- Fat: 20g
- Carbohydrates: 30g
- Fiber: 6g

Serves: 8

Cooking Time: 60 minutes

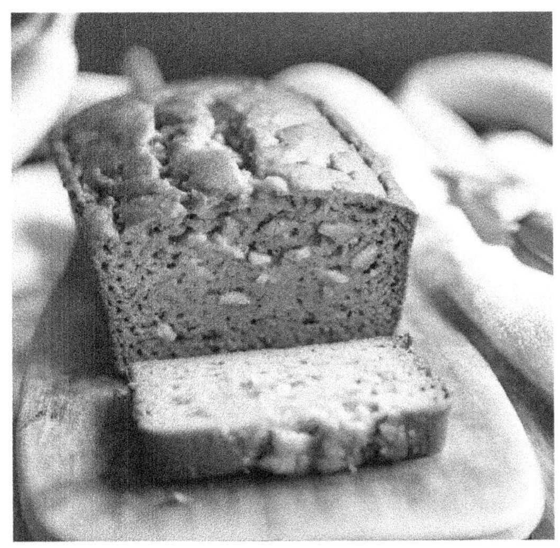

22. Coconut Almond Porridge

Ingredients:
- 1/3 cup almond flour
- 1/4 cup shredded coonut
- 2 tablespoons ground flaxseed
- 1 cup coconut milk
- 1/2 teaspoon cinnamon
- 1 tablespoon maple syrup or honey (optional)
- Fresh berries or nuts for topping

Instructions:
1. In a small pot, combine the almond flour, shredded coconut, ground flaxseed, and coconut milk. Mix well.
2. Cook over medium heat, stirring constantly to prevent clumping, until the mixture thickens, usually about 5-7 minutes.
3. Stir in the cinnamon and maple syrup or honey if desired, blending well.
4. Once cooked to a porridge-like consistency, remove from heat and let it sit for a minute to thicken further.
5. Serve warm, topped with fresh berries or nuts of your choice.

Nutritional Info (per serving):
- Calories: ~300
- Protein: 6g
- Fat: 25g
- Carbohydrates: 15g
- Fiber: 6g

Serves: 2

Cooking Time: 10 minutes

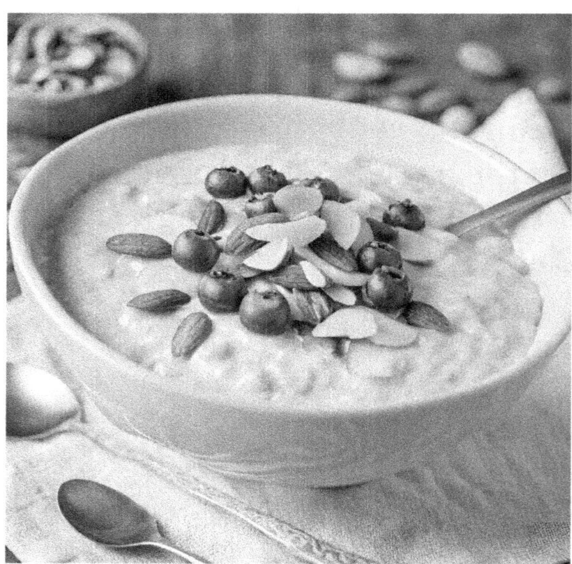

POULTRY & MEAT RECIPES

1. Ethiopian Doro Wat
Ingredients:
- 2 lbs chicken thighs, skinless
- 2 tablespoons olive oil
- 2 large onions, finely chopped
- 4 cloves garlic, minced
- 1 tablespoon ginger, minced
- 2 tablespoons paprika
- 1 tablespoon berbere spice mix (or adjust to taste)
- 1 can (14 oz) diced tomatoes
- 4 hard-boiled eggs
- Salt to taste
- 1/2 cup chicken broth

Instructions:
1. In a large pot, heat olive oil over medium heat. Add onions and cook until soft, about 5 minutes. Add garlic and ginger; cook for another 2 minutes.
2. Stir in paprika and berbere spice, cooking for 1 minute until fragrant.
3. Add the chicken thighs and diced tomatoes, ensuring the chicken is well-coated with the spices. Season with salt.
4. Pour in chicken broth, cover, and simmer on low heat for 45 minutes.
5. Gently add hard-boiled eggs to the pot in the last 10 minutes of cooking.

Nutritional Info (per serving):
- Calories: ~450
- Protein: 35g
- Fat: 25g
- Carbohydrates: 15g
- Fiber: 4g

Serves: 6
Cooking Time: 60 minutes

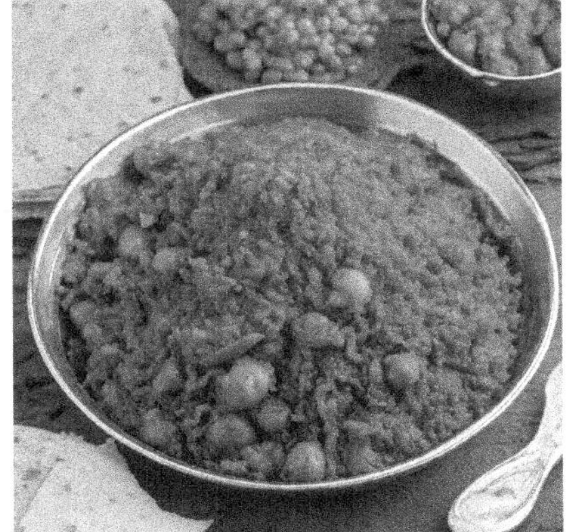

2. Irish Beef Stew

Ingredients:

- 2 lbs beef stew meat, cubed
- 3 tablespoons olive oil
- 3 large carrots, chopped
- 2 large parsnips, chopped
- 1 onion, chopped
- 3 cloves garlic, minced
- 4 cups beef broth
- 1 cup Guinness beer (optional, replace with more broth for Hashimoto's-friendly version)
- 2 tablespoons tomato paste
- 1 teaspoon thyme
- Salt and pepper to taste
- 2 tablespoons arrowroot powder (for thickening, optional)

Instructions:

1. In a large pot, heat 1 tablespoon olive oil over medium-high heat. Brown the beef in batches, then set aside.
2. Reduce heat to medium, add remaining oil, and cook onions, carrots, and parsnips until slightly softened.
3. Add garlic, tomato paste, and thyme; cook for 1 minute.
4. Return beef to the pot. Add beef broth (and beer if using, though not recommended for Hashimoto's). Season with salt and pepper.
5. Cover, reduce heat to low, and simmer for 1.5 to 2 hours, until beef is tender.
6. If desired, mix arrowroot powder with water and stir into stew to thicken.

Nutritional Info (per serving):

- Calories: ~500
- Protein: 40g
- Fat: 30g
- Carbohydrates: 20g
- Fiber: 4g

Serves: 6

Cooking Time: 2.5 hours

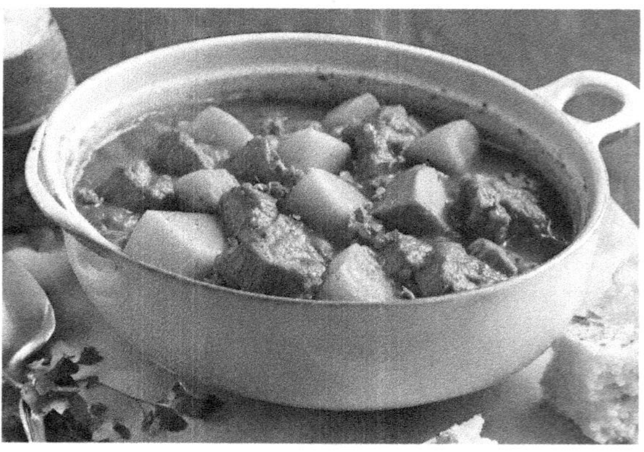

3. Vietnamese Shaking Beef (Bò Lúc Lắc)

Ingredients:

- 2 lbs sirloin steak, cut into 1-inch cubes
- 2 tablespoons olive oil
- 1 tablespoon soy sauce (gluten-free)
- 1 tablespoon fish sauce
- 1 tablespoon oyster sauce (gluten-free)
- 2 cloves garlic, minced
- 1 teaspoon sugar or honey
- 1 red onion, sliced
- 2 scallions, chopped
- 1/2 teaspoon black pepper
- Lettuce leaves and tomato slices for serving

Instructions:

1. Marinate beef with soy sauce, fish sauce, oyster sauce, garlic, and sugar for at least 30 minutes.
2. Heat olive oil in a wok or large skillet over high heat. Add beef and sear quickly on all sides.
3. Add red onion and scallions, shaking the pan (hence "shaking beef"), and cook for an additional 2 minutes.
4. Serve immediately on a bed of lettuce and tomato slices, sprinkled with black pepper.

Nutritional Info (per serving):

- Calories: ~350
- Protein: 40g
- Fat: 20g
- Carbohydrates: 5g
- Fiber: 1g

Serves: 4

Cooking Time: 40 minutes (including marinating time)

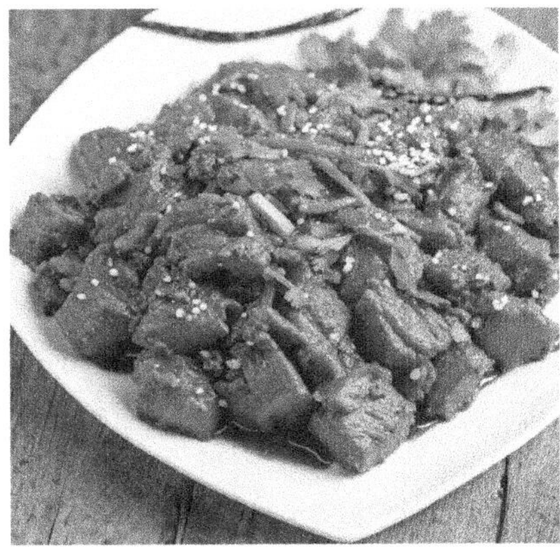

4. Peruvian Roast Chicken
Ingredients:
- 1 whole chicken (about 4 lbs), giblets removed
- 2 tablespoons olive oil
- 2 tablespoons lime juice
- 4 cloves garlic, minced
- 1 tablespoon ground cumin
- 1 tablespoon smoked paprika
- 1 teaspoon dried oregano
- 1 teaspoon salt
- 1/2 teaspoon black pepper
- 1/2 teaspoon ground turmeric

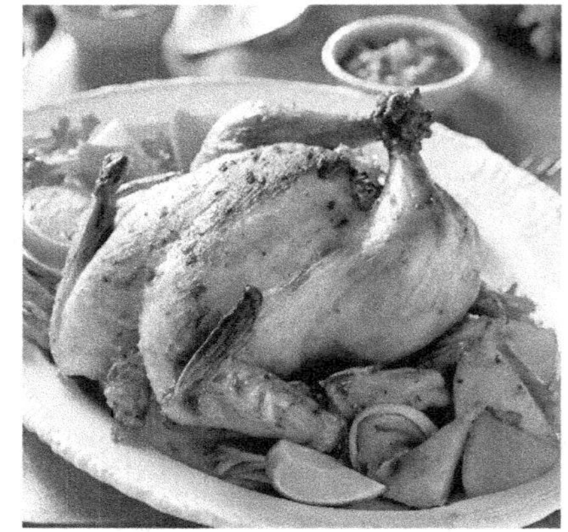

Instructions:
1. Preheat your oven to 375°F (190°C).
2. In a small bowl, mix together olive oil, lime juice, garlic, cumin, paprika, oregano, salt, pepper, and turmeric to create a marinade.
3. Rub the marinade all over the chicken, inside and out. Let it marinate for at least 30 minutes, or overnight in the fridge for deeper flavor.
4. Place the chicken in a roasting pan, breast side up. Roast in the preheated oven for about 1 hour and 20 minutes, or until the internal temperature reaches 165°F (74°C) and the juices run clear.
5. Let the chicken rest for 10 minutes before carving. Serve with your choice of sides.

Nutritional Info (per serving):
- Calories: ~400 (varies with portion size)
- Protein: 35g
- Fat: 25g
- Carbohydrates: 2g
- Fiber: 0.5g

Serves: 4-6

Cooking Time: 1 hour 50 minutes (including marinating and resting time)

5. Lebanese Garlic Chicken

Ingredients:

- 2 lbs chicken thighs, bone-in, skin-on
- 1/4 cup olive oil
- 10 cloves garlic, minced
- 1/4 cup lemon juice
- 1 teaspoon salt
- 1/2 teaspoon black pepper
- 1 teaspoon paprika
- 1/2 teaspoon ground cumin
- Fresh parsley for garnish

Instructions:

1. Preheat the oven to 400°F (200°C).
2. In a bowl, combine olive oil, minced garlic, lemon juice, salt, pepper, paprika, and cumin to create a marinade.
3. Toss the chicken thighs in the marinade until well coated. Arrange them in a single layer in a baking dish.
4. Roast in the preheated oven for 35-40 minutes, or until the chicken is cooked through and the skin is crispy.
5. Garnish with fresh parsley before serving.

Nutritional Info (per serving):

- Calories: ~450
- Protein: 30g
- Fat: 35g
- Carbohydrates: 3g
- Fiber: 0.5g

Serves: 4

Cooking Time: 45 minutes

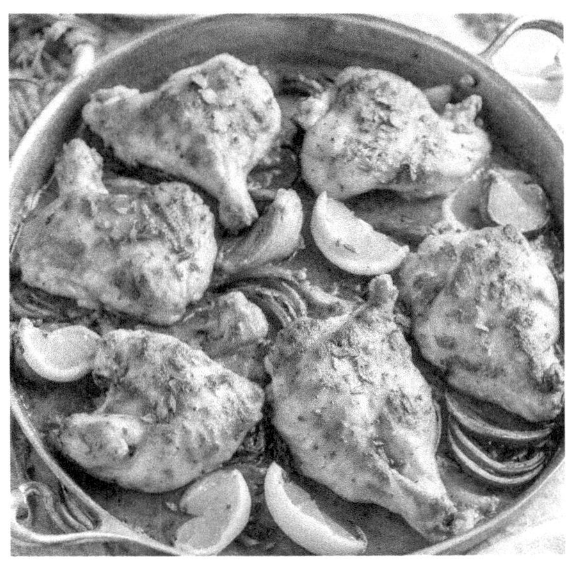

6. Hungarian Beef Goulash

Ingredients:

- 2 lbs beef chuck, cut into 1-inch cubes
- 3 tablespoons olive oil
- 2 large onions, chopped
- 3 cloves garlic, minced
- 2 tablespoons Hungarian paprika
- 1 teaspoon caraway seeds
- 1 can (14 oz) diced tomatoes
- 2 cups beef broth
- 2 red bell peppers, chopped
- 2 carrots, sliced
- 1 teaspoon salt
- 1/2 teaspoon black pepper

Instructions:

1. Heat 1 tablespoon of olive oil in a large pot over medium-high heat. Brown the beef in batches, then set aside.
2. Reduce heat to medium, add remaining olive oil, and sauté onions and garlic until soft.
3. Return the beef to the pot, stir in paprika and caraway seeds until well coated. Add diced tomatoes and beef broth.
4. Bring to a simmer, then cover and cook on low heat for 1.5 hours.
5. Add red bell peppers and carrots, cook for another 30 minutes, or until vegetables and beef are tender.
6. Season with salt and pepper to taste. Serve hot.

Nutritional Info (per serving):

- Calories: ~500
- Protein: 40g
- Fat: 30g
- Carbohydrates: 15g
- Fiber: 4g

Serves: 6

Cooking Time: 2 hours 15 minutes

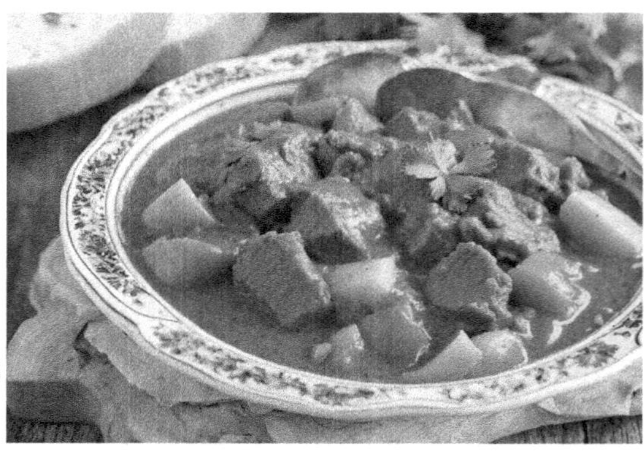

7. Sicilian Chicken Soup

Ingredients:

- 1 lb chicken breast, cubed
- 2 tablespoons olive oil
- 1 onion, chopped
- 2 carrots, diced
- 2 celery stalks, diced
- 3 cloves garlic, minced
- 1 can (14 oz) diced tomatoes
- 6 cups chicken broth
- 1 cup chopped kale
- 1/2 cup fresh basil, chopped
- Salt and pepper to taste

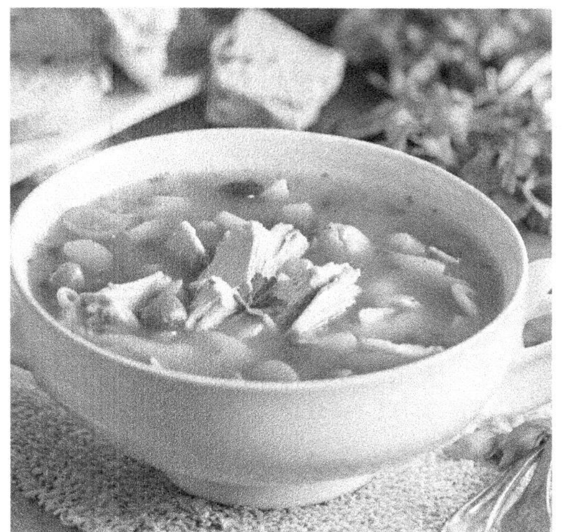

Instructions:

1. In a large pot, heat olive oil over medium heat. Add the onion, carrots, and celery, cooking until they begin to soften, about 5 minutes.
2. Add the garlic and cubed chicken breast to the pot. Cook until the chicken is no longer pink on the outside, approximately 5-7 minutes.
3. Stir in the diced tomatoes and chicken broth. Bring to a simmer.
4. Reduce the heat to low and let the soup cook, covered, for about 25 minutes to allow the flavors to meld.
5. Add the chopped kale and fresh basil in the last 5 minutes of cooking. Season with salt and pepper to taste.
6. Serve the soup hot, adjusting seasoning as needed.

Nutritional Info (per serving):

- Calories: ~250
- Protein: 25g
- Fat: 10g
- Carbohydrates: 15g
- Fiber: 3g

Serves: 6

Cooking Time: 40 minutes

8. Thai Basil Chicken

Ingredients:

- 2 lbs chicken breast, thinly sliced
- 2 tablespoons olive oil
- 3 cloves garlic, minced
- 1 small red chili, finely sliced (adjust to taste)
- 2 tablespoons soy sauce (gluten-free)
- 1 tablespoon fish sauce
- 1 teaspoon honey or coconut sugar
- 1 cup fresh basil leaves
- Salt to taste

Instructions:

1. Heat olive oil in a large skillet over medium-high heat. Add garlic and chili, sautéing until fragrant.
2. Add the chicken slices, stirring until they start to brown.
3. Stir in soy sauce, fish sauce, and honey, cooking until the chicken is fully cooked.
4. Remove from heat and stir in fresh basil leaves until wilted. Season with salt if needed.
5. Serve hot over steamed rice or a bed of vegetables for a low-carb option.

Nutritional Info (per serving):

- Calories: ~300
- Protein: 44g
- Fat: 12g
- Carbohydrates: 5g
- Fiber: 1g

Serves: 4

Cooking Time: 20 minutes

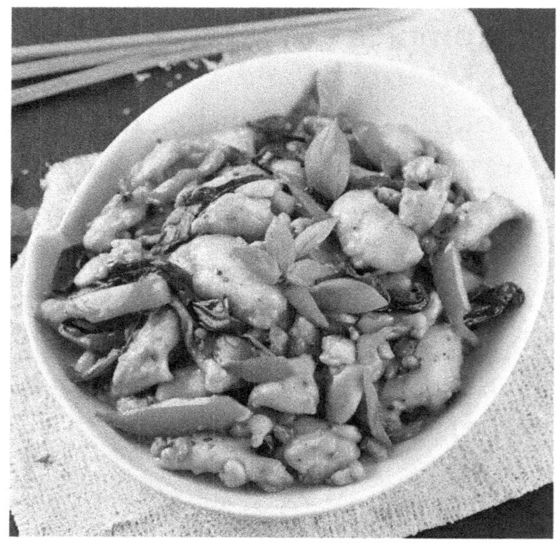

9. Cuban Mojo Pork

Ingredients:

- 2 lbs pork shoulder, cut into chunks
- 1/4 cup olive oil
- 1/4 cup orange juice
- 2 tablespoons lime juice
- 6 cloves garlic, minced
- 1 teaspoon cumin
- 1 teaspoon oregano
- 1 teaspoon salt
- 1/2 teaspoon black pepper
- 1 small onion, sliced
- 1/4 cup fresh cilantro, chopped

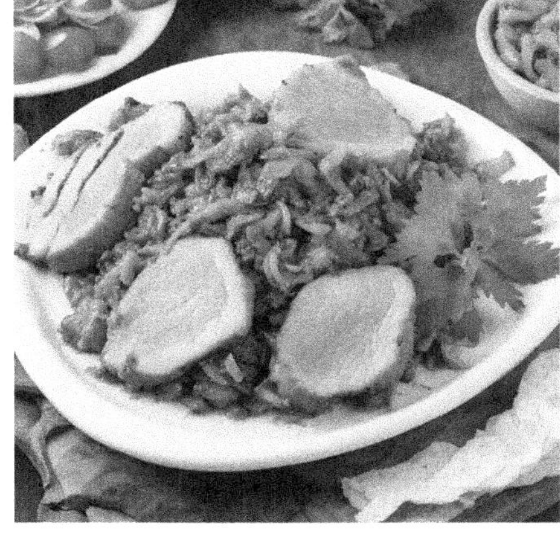

Instructions:

1. In a bowl, whisk together olive oil, orange juice, lime juice, garlic, cumin, oregano, salt, and pepper to create the mojo marinade.
2. Pour the marinade over the pork chunks in a large zip-lock bag. Add the sliced onion. Marinate in the refrigerator for at least 2 hours, or overnight.
3. Preheat the oven to 325°F (163°C). Place pork and marinade in a roasting pan.
4. Cover and roast for 2.5 to 3 hours, until the pork is tender and shreds easily.
5. Garnish with fresh cilantro before serving.

Nutritional Info (per serving):

- Calories: ~400
- Protein: 35g
- Fat: 27g
- Carbohydrates: 5g
- Fiber: 1g

Serves: 6

Cooking Time: 3 hours 15 minutes (including marinating time)

10. Turkish Chicken Kebabs

Ingredients:

- 2 lbs chicken breast, cut into cubes
- 2 tablespoons olive oil
- 2 tablespoons yogurt (dairy-free if necessary)
- 4 cloves garlic, minced
- 1 tablespoon paprika
- 1 teaspoon cumin
- 1/2 teaspoon cinnamon
- Salt and pepper to taste
- 1 lemon, for serving

Instructions:

1. In a large bowl, mix olive oil, yogurt, garlic, paprika, cumin, cinnamon, salt, and pepper. Add the chicken cubes, ensuring they are well coated. Marinate for at least 1 hour, or overnight.
2. Preheat the grill to medium-high heat. Thread the chicken onto skewers.
3. Grill for 10-15 minutes, turning occasionally, until the chicken is cooked through.
4. Serve with lemon wedges on the side.

Nutritional Info (per serving):

- Calories: ~300
- Protein: 44g
- Fat: 12g
- Carbohydrates: 3g
- Fiber: 0.5g

Serves: 4

Cooking Time: 25 minutes (including marinating time)

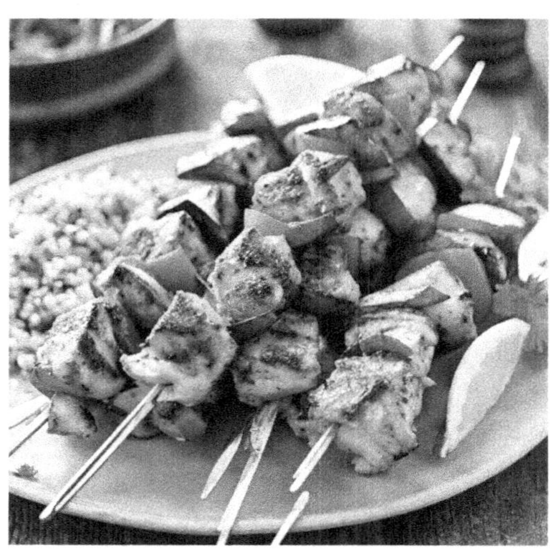

11. Paleo Beef Stroganoff

Ingredients:

- 2 lbs beef sirloin, thinly sliced
- 2 tablespoons olive oil
- 1 onion, thinly sliced
- 2 cloves garlic, minced
- 8 oz mushrooms, sliced
- 1 cup beef broth
- 1 cup coconut cream
- 1 tablespoon Dijon mustard
- Salt and pepper to taste
- Fresh parsley for garnish

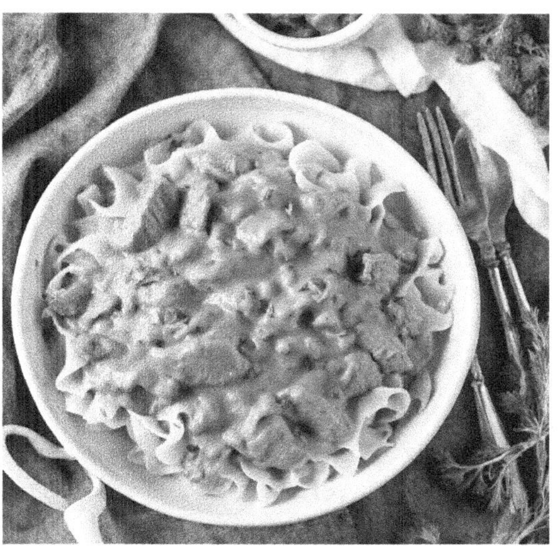

Instructions:

1. In a large skillet, heat olive oil over medium-high heat. Add beef slices and cook until browned. Remove from the skillet and set aside.
2. In the same skillet, add another tablespoon of olive oil if necessary. Sauté onion and garlic until soft. Add mushrooms and cook until they release their moisture.
3. Return the beef to the skillet. Add beef broth, coconut cream, and Dijon mustard.
4. Stir well and bring to a simmer. Reduce heat and cook for an additional 5-7 minutes, until the sauce thickens slightly.
5. Season with salt and pepper to taste. Garnish with fresh parsley before serving.
6. Serve over cooked spaghetti squash or zucchini noodles for a complete paleo meal.

Nutritional Info (per serving):

- Calories: ~450
- Protein: 35g
- Fat: 30g
- Carbohydrates: 8g
- Fiber: 1g

Serves: 4

Cooking Time: 30 minutes

12. Chicken Tikka Masala

Ingredients:

- 2 lbs chicken breast, cut into chunks
- 1 cup plain yogurt (dairy-free if needed)
- 2 tablespoons lemon juice
- 2 teaspoons turmeric powder
- 2 teaspoons garam masala
- 1 teaspoon cumin
- 1 teaspoon paprika
- 1 tablespoon grated ginger
- 3 cloves garlic, minced
- Salt to taste
- 2 tablespoons olive oil
- 1 large onion, finely chopped
- 1 can (14 oz) crushed tomatoes
- 1 cup coconut cream
- Fresh cilantro for garnish

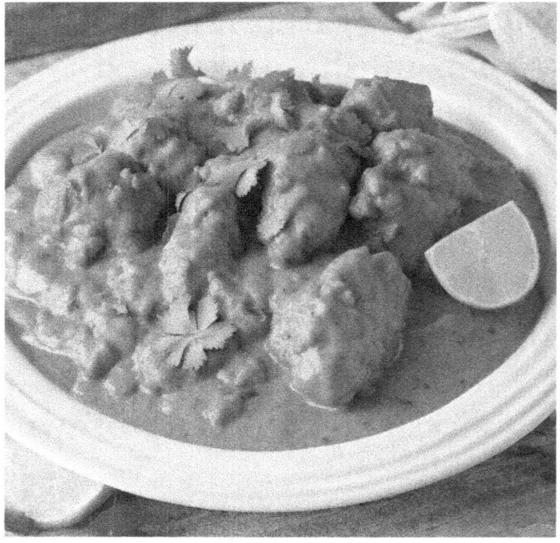

Instructions:

1. In a bowl, mix together yogurt, lemon juice, turmeric, garam masala, cumin, paprika, ginger, garlic, and salt. Add the chicken chunks, ensuring they are well coated. Marinate for at least 1 hour, or overnight in the refrigerator.
2. Heat olive oil in a large skillet over medium heat. Add the marinated chicken and cook until browned. Remove chicken and set aside.
3. In the same skillet, add the onion and sauté until translucent. Add the crushed tomatoes and bring to a simmer.
4. Return the chicken to the skillet, cover, and simmer for 20 minutes.
5. Stir in coconut cream and simmer for an additional 10 minutes, until the sauce thickens.
6. Garnish with fresh cilantro and serve with cauliflower rice for a low-carb option.

Nutritional Info (per serving):

- Calories: ~400 Protein: 40g Fat: 22g
- Carbohydrates: 12g
- Fiber: 3g

Serves: 4

Cooking Time: 1 hour 40 minutes (including marinating time)

13. Mediterranean Lamb Kebabs

Ingredients:

- 2 lbs lamb shoulder, cut into 1-inch cubes
- 1/4 cup olive oil
- 2 tablespoons lemon juice
- 3 cloves garlic, minced
- 1 teaspoon rosemary, chopped
- 1 teaspoon thyme, chopped
- Salt and pepper to taste

Instructions:

1. In a bowl, combine olive oil, lemon juice, garlic, rosemary, thyme, salt, and pepper. Add the lamb cubes and toss to coat. Marinate for at least 2 hours, or overnight in the refrigerator.
2. Preheat grill to medium-high heat. Thread the lamb onto skewers.
3. Grill for 10-12 minutes, turning occasionally, until the lamb is cooked to your liking.
4. Serve hot, garnished with fresh herbs or a side of tzatziki sauce.

Nutritional Info (per serving):

- Calories: ~400
- Protein: 35g
- Fat: 28g
- Carbohydrates: 2g
- Fiber: 0g

Serves: 4

Cooking Time: 2 hours 20 minutes (including marinating time)

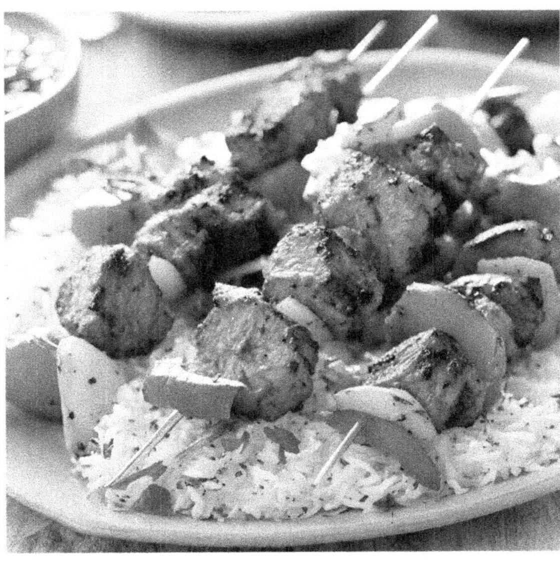

14. Chicken Shawarma Salad

Ingredients:

- 2 lbs chicken thighs, boneless and skinless
- 2 tablespoons olive oil
- 1 tablespoon shawarma spice blend
- Juice of 1 lemon
- Salt to taste
- Mixed salad greens
- Cherry tomatoes, halved
- Cucumber, sliced
- Red onion, thinly sliced
- Tahini dressing

Instructions:

1. In a bowl, mix olive oil, shawarma spice, lemon juice, and salt. Add chicken thighs and ensure they're well coated. Marinate for at least 1 hour or overnight.
2. Preheat the oven to 375°F (190°C) or prepare a grill. Cook the chicken until it's fully done, about 25-30 minutes in the oven or 10-15 minutes on the grill, turning halfway through.
3. Let the chicken rest for a few minutes, then slice it thinly.
4. Assemble the salad with mixed greens, cherry tomatoes, cucumber, and red onion. Top with sliced chicken and drizzle with tahini dressing.

Nutritional Info (per serving):

- Calories: ~350 Protein: 40g Fat: 18g Carbohydrates: 8g
- Fiber: 2g

Serves: 4

Cooking Time: 1 hour 35 minutes (including marinating time)

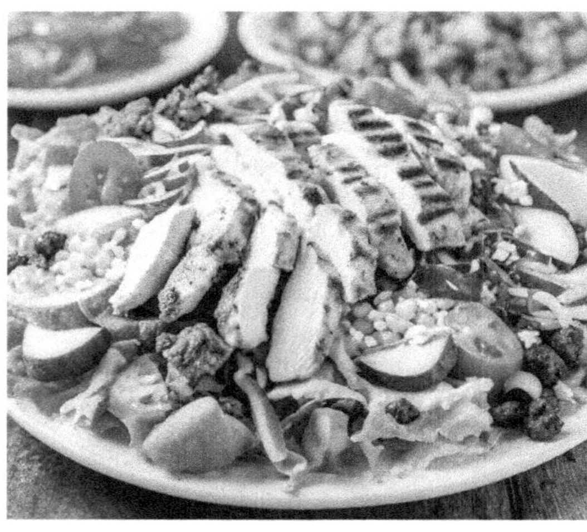

15. Beef Bulgogi

Ingredients:

- 2 lbs thinly sliced ribeye steak
- 1/4 cup soy sauce (gluten-free)
- 2 tablespoons sesame oil
- 2 tablespoons brown sugar or honey
- 4 cloves garlic, minced
- 1 pear, grated (for tenderizing and sweetness)
- 2 green onions, chopped
- 1 tablespoon sesame seeds
- 1/2 teaspoon black pepper

Instructions:

1. In a bowl, combine soy sauce, sesame oil, brown sugar or honey, garlic, grated pear, green onions, sesame seeds, and black pepper to make the marinade.
2. Add the beef slices to the marinade, ensuring each piece is well coated. Marinate for at least 1 hour, or overnight for best flavor.
3. Heat a grill pan or skillet over medium-high heat. Cook the beef in batches, 1-2 minutes per side, until browned and slightly charred.
4. Serve hot with steamed rice and a side of kimchi or a fresh salad.

Nutritional Info (per serving):

- Calories: ~450
- Protein: 40g
- Fat: 25g
- Carbohydrates: 15g
- Fiber: 1g

Serves: 4

Cooking Time: 1 hour 20 minutes (including marinating time)

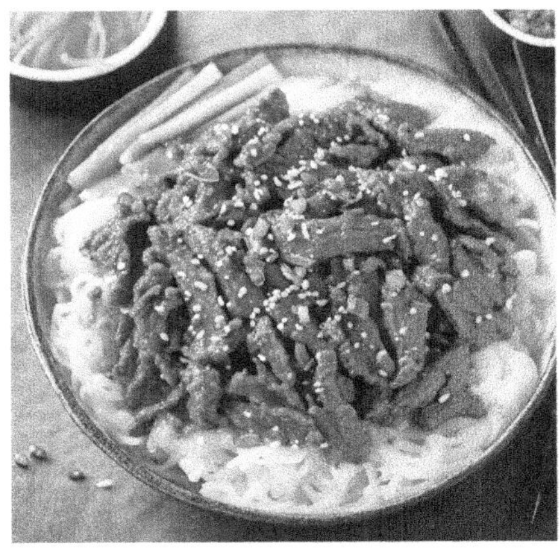

16. Jamaican Jerk Chicken
Ingredients:
- 2 lbs chicken thighs, bone-in, skin-on
- 1/4 cup olive oil
- 1/4 cup soy sauce (gluten-free)
- 1/4 cup vinegar
- 2 tablespoons brown sugar or honey
- 1 Scotch bonnet pepper, chopped (adjust to taste)
- 2 teaspoons allspice
- 2 teaspoons thyme
- 4 cloves garlic, minced
- 1 teaspoon cinnamon
- 1 teaspoon nutmeg
- Salt to taste

Instructions:
1. Blend olive oil, soy sauce, vinegar, brown sugar or honey, Scotch bonnet pepper, allspice, thyme, garlic, cinnamon, and nutmeg to create a jerk marinade.
2. Place chicken in a large bowl or zip-lock bag and pour the marinade over it. Ensure each piece is coated well. Marinate for at least 4 hours, preferably overnight.
3. Preheat grill to medium-high heat. Grill the chicken, turning occasionally, until it is cooked through and the skin is crispy, about 25-30 minutes.
4. Serve hot with rice and peas or a fresh salad.

Nutritional Info (per serving):
- Calories: ~400
- Protein: 35g
- Fat: 25g
- Carbohydrates: 10g
- Fiber: 1g

Serves: 4
Cooking Time: 4 hours 30 minutes (including marinating time)

17. Italian Herb Chicken Thighs

Ingredients:

- 2 lbs chicken thighs, bone-in, skin-on
- 2 tablespoons olive oil
- 2 tablespoons Italian seasoning (blend of oregano, basil, thyme, rosemary)
- 4 cloves garlic, minced
- Salt and pepper to taste
- 1 lemon, sliced for garnish
- Fresh parsley, chopped for garnish

Instructions:

1. Preheat the oven to 400°F (200°C).
2. In a bowl, combine olive oil, Italian seasoning, minced garlic, salt, and pepper. Rub this mixture all over the chicken thighs.
3. Arrange chicken thighs on a baking sheet and place lemon slices around them.
4. Roast in the preheated oven for 35-40 minutes, or until the chicken is golden on the outside and reaches an internal temperature of 165°F (74°C).
5. Garnish with fresh parsley before serving.

Nutritional Info (per serving):

- Calories: ~350
- Protein: 30g
- Fat: 25g
- Carbohydrates: 2g
- Fiber: 0.5g

Serves: 4
Cooking Time: 45 minutes

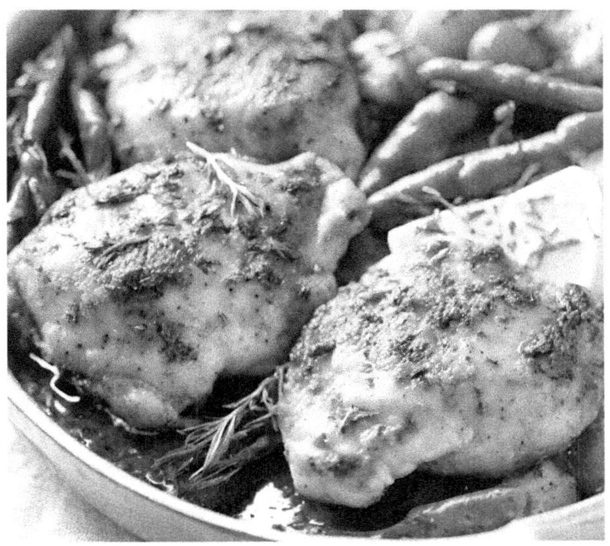

18. Asian Turkey Lettuce Wraps

Ingredients:

- 1 lb ground turkey
- 1 tablespoon olive oil
- 2 cloves garlic, minced
- 1 inch fresh ginger, grated
- 1 red bell pepper, diced
- 1/2 cup carrots, shredded
- 1/4 cup green onions, chopped
- 2 tablespoons soy sauce (gluten-free)
- 1 tablespoon hoisin sauce (gluten-free, if available)
- 1 teaspoon sesame oil
- Salt and pepper to taste
- 1 head of lettuce, leaves separated (e.g., iceberg or butter lettuce)
- Optional garnishes: chopped peanuts, cilantro

Instructions:

1. Heat olive oil in a large skillet over medium heat. Add garlic and ginger, sautéing until fragrant.
2. Add ground turkey to the skillet, breaking it apart with a spoon. Cook until browned.
3. Stir in red bell pepper and carrots, cooking for a few minutes until slightly soft.
4. Mix in soy sauce, hoisin sauce, sesame oil, and green onions. Season with salt and pepper. Cook for another 2-3 minutes.
5. Serve the turkey mixture in lettuce leaves, garnished with peanuts and cilantro if desired.

Nutritional Info (per serving):

- Calories: ~250
- Protein: 22g
- Fat: 15g
- Carbohydrates: 8g
- Fiber: 2g

Serves: 4

Cooking Time: 20 minutes

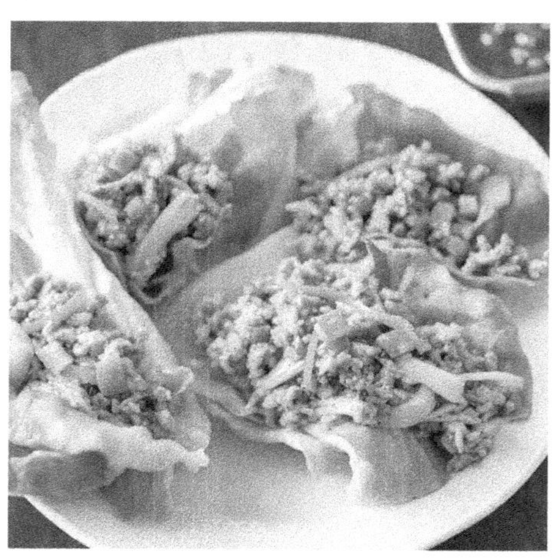

19. Chicken Cacciatore

Ingredients:

- 2 lbs chicken thighs, bone-in, skin-on
- 1 tablespoon olive oil
- 1 onion, sliced
- 2 bell peppers, sliced
- 2 cloves garlic, minced
- 1 can (28 oz) diced tomatoes
- 1/2 cup chicken broth
- 1 teaspoon dried oregano
- 1 teaspoon dried basil
- Salt and pepper to taste
- Fresh parsley for garnish

Instructions:

1. In a large skillet, heat olive oil over medium-high heat. Season chicken with salt and pepper, then brown on both sides. Remove from skillet.
2. In the same skillet, add onions, bell peppers, and garlic. Sauté until softened.
3. Return chicken to the skillet. Add diced tomatoes, chicken broth, oregano, and basil.
4. Cover and simmer on low heat for 45 minutes, until chicken is cooked through.
5. Garnish with fresh parsley before serving.

Nutritional Info (per serving):

- Calories: ~400
- Protein: 30g
- Fat: 25g
- Carbohydrates: 10g
- Fiber: 3g

Serves: 4

Cooking Time: 1 hour

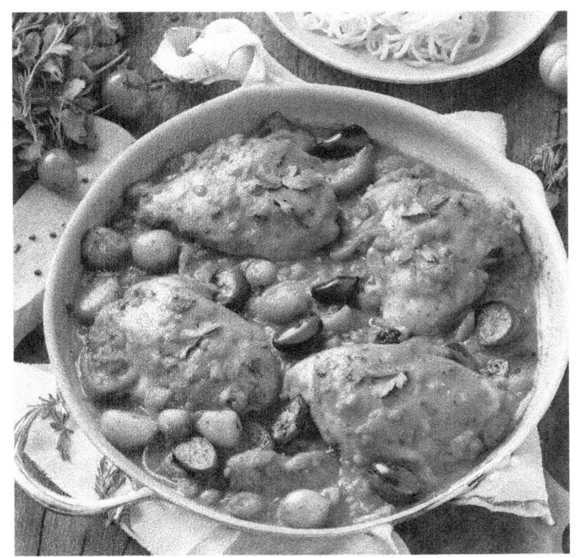

20. Herb-Roasted Turkey Breast

Ingredients:

- 1 bone-in turkey breast (about 3 lbs)
- 2 tablespoons olive oil
- 1 tablespoon fresh rosemary, minced
- 1 tablespoon fresh thyme, minced
- 2 cloves garlic, minced
- Salt and pepper to taste

Instructions:

1. Preheat oven to 350°F (175°C).
2. In a small bowl, mix olive oil, rosemary, thyme, garlic, salt, and pepper. Rub this mixture all over the turkey breast.
3. Place turkey breast in a roasting pan and roast for 1.5 to 2 hours, or until the internal temperature reaches 165°F (74°C).
4. Let rest for 10 minutes before slicing.

Nutritional Info (per serving):

- Calories: ~300
- Protein: 55g
- Fat: 7g
- Carbohydrates: 0g
- Fiber: 0g

Serves: 6

Cooking Time: 2 hours 10 minutes (including resting time)

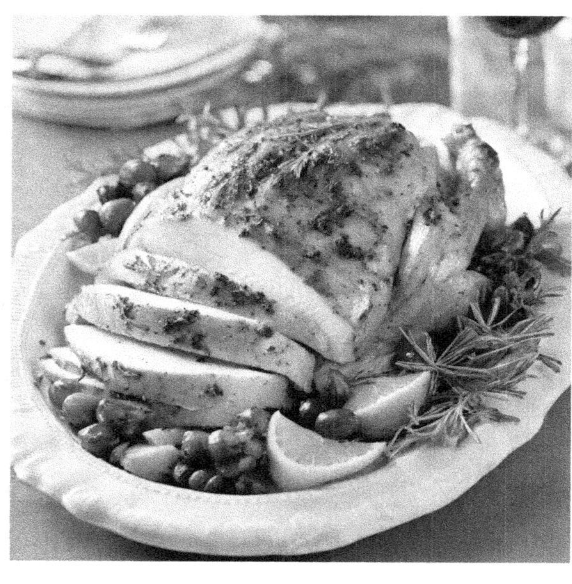

21. Greek Lamb Meatballs

Ingredients:

- 1 lb ground lamb
- 1/4 cup almond flour
- 1 egg
- 2 cloves garlic, minced
- 2 tablespoons fresh mint, chopped
- 1 tablespoon dried oregano
- Salt and pepper to taste
- Olive oil for frying

Instructions:

1. In a bowl, combine ground lamb, almond flour, egg, garlic, mint, oregano, salt, and pepper. Mix until well combined.
2. Form the mixture into small meatballs.
3. Heat olive oil in a skillet over medium heat. Fry the meatballs until browned and cooked through, about 4-5 minutes per side.
4. Serve hot with tzatziki sauce and a side of Greek salad.

Nutritional Info (per serving):

- Calories: ~350
- Protein: 22g
- Fat: 27g
- Carbohydrates: 3g
- Fiber: 1g

Serves: 4

Cooking Time: 30 minutes

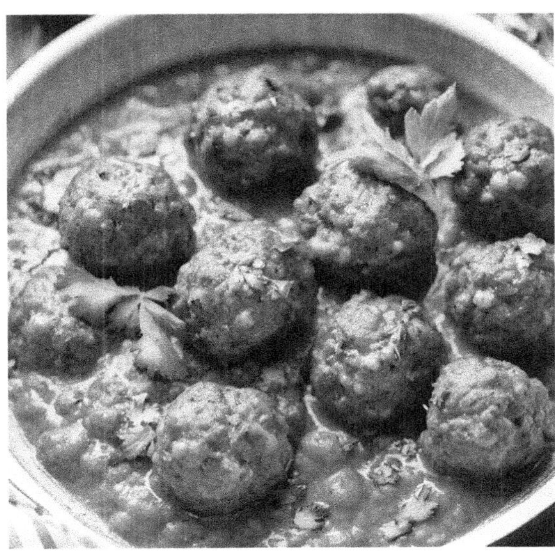

22. Indian Chicken Curry

Ingredients:

- 2 lbs chicken thighs, cut into pieces
- 2 tablespoons coconut oil
- 1 large onion, finely chopped
- 3 cloves garlic, minced
- 1 inch ginger, grated
- 2 tablespoons curry powder
- 1 teaspoon turmeric
- 1 can (14 oz) coconut milk
- 1 can (14 oz) diced tomatoes
- Salt and pepper to taste
- Fresh cilantro for garnish

Instructions:

1. Heat coconut oil in a large skillet over medium heat. Add onion, garlic, and ginger, sautéing until onion is translucent.
2. Add curry powder and turmeric, stirring until fragrant.
3. Add chicken pieces to the skillet, browning on all sides.
4. Pour in coconut milk and diced tomatoes. Season with salt and pepper.
5. Cover and simmer on low heat for 30 minutes, until chicken is cooked through.
6. Garnish with fresh cilantro before serving. Serve with cauliflower rice or steamed vegetables for a complete meal.

Nutritional Info (per serving):

- Calories: ~450
- Protein: 30g
- Fat: 35g
- Carbohydrates: 8g
- Fiber: 2g

Serves: 4

Cooking Time: 45 minutes

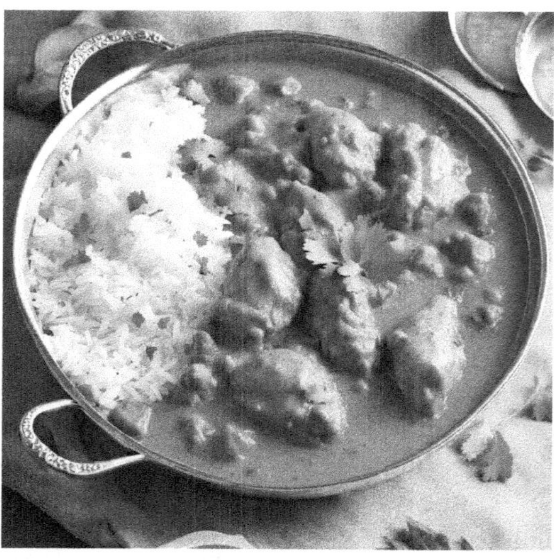

23. Moroccan Lamb Tagine

Ingredients:

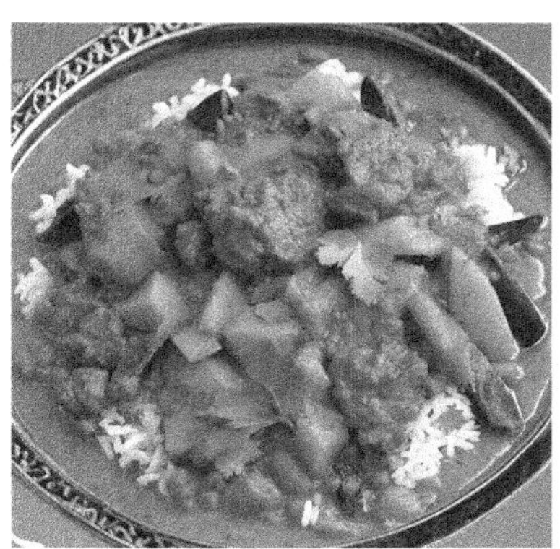

- 2 lbs lamb shoulder, cut into chunks
- 2 tablespoons olive oil
- 1 large onion, chopped
- 3 cloves garlic, minced
- 1 teaspoon ground cumin
- 1 teaspoon ground cinnamon
- 1/2 teaspoon ground ginger
- 1/2 teaspoon paprika
- 1/4 teaspoon saffron threads (optional)
- 2 cups beef or chicken broth
- 1 can (14 oz) diced tomatoes
- 1 cup dried apricots, chopped
- Salt and pepper to taste
- Fresh parsley and toasted almonds for garnish

Instructions:

1. In a large pot or tagine, heat olive oil over medium heat. Add the lamb, browning on all sides. Remove lamb and set aside.
2. In the same pot, add onion and garlic, cooking until softened.
3. Return lamb to the pot, adding cumin, cinnamon, ginger, paprika, and saffron. Stir to coat the lamb.
4. Add broth and diced tomatoes, bringing to a simmer. Cover and cook on low heat for 1.5 hours.
5. Add dried apricots, continuing to simmer for another 30 minutes, until lamb is tender and sauce has thickened.
6. Season with salt and pepper. Garnish with parsley and toasted almonds before serving.

Nutritional Info (per serving):

- Calories: ~500
- Protein: 40g
- Fat: 30g
- Carbohydrates: 25g
- Fiber: 5g

Serves: 4

Cooking Time: 2 hours 15 minutes

24. Beef Stir-Fry

Ingredients:

- 1 lb beef sirloin, thinly sliced
- 2 tablespoons soy sauce (gluten-free)
- 1 tablespoon sesame oil
- 1 tablespoon cornstarch or arrowroot powder
- 2 tablespoons coconut oil
- 1 bell pepper, sliced
- 1 onion, sliced
- 2 cloves garlic, minced
- 1 tablespoon fresh ginger, grated
- 1/2 cup beef broth
- 1 tablespoon hoisin sauce (gluten-free, if available)
- Salt and pepper to taste
- Sesame seeds and green onions for garnish

Instructions:

1. In a bowl, marinate beef slices in soy sauce, sesame oil, and cornstarch for at least 15 minutes.
2. Heat coconut oil in a large skillet or wok over high heat. Add beef and stir-fry until browned. Remove beef and set aside.
3. In the same skillet, add more oil if necessary. Stir-fry bell pepper, onion, garlic, and ginger until vegetables are just tender.
4. Return beef to the skillet. Add beef broth and hoisin sauce, cooking until the sauce has thickened.
5. Season with salt and pepper. Garnish with sesame seeds and green onions before serving.

Nutritional Info (per serving):

- Calories: ~350
- Protein: 25g
- Fat: 22g
- Carbohydrates: 10g
- Fiber: 2g

Serves: 4

Cooking Time: 30 minutes

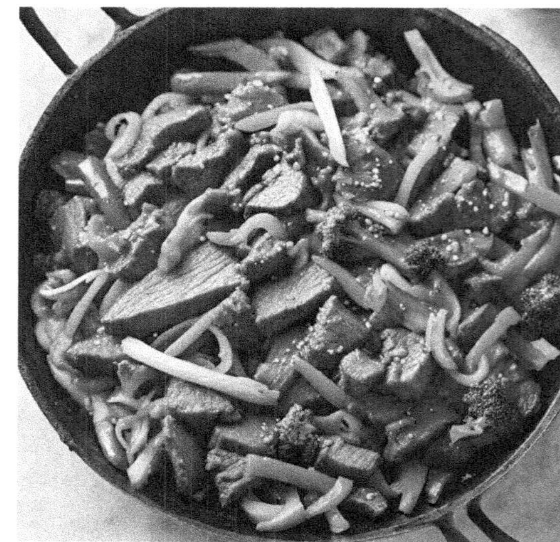

Fish & Seafood Recipes

1. Grilled Salmon with Avocado Salsa
Ingredients:

- 4 salmon fillets (about 6 oz each)
- 2 tablespoons olive oil
- Salt and pepper to taste
- 2 avocados, diced
- 1 small red onion, finely chopped
- 1 toma
- Juice
- 1/4 cu
- 1 jalap

Instructi

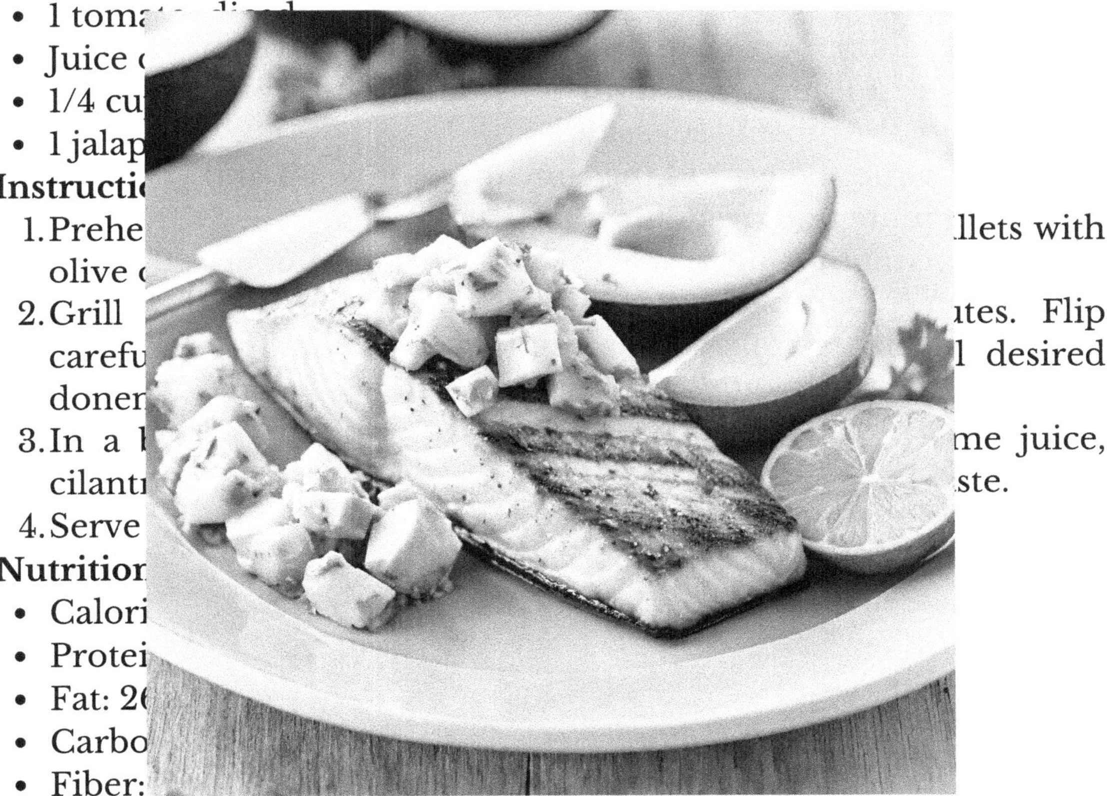

1. Prehe…llets with olive
2. Grill…tes. Flip carefu…l desired doner
3. In a…me juice, cilantr…ste.
4. Serve

Nutritior

- Calori
- Protei
- Fat: 2(
- Carbo
- Fiber:

Serves: 4
Cooking Time: 15 minutes

2. Shrimp Zoodle Alfredo

Ingredients:

- 1 lb shrimp, peeled and deveined
- 4 medium zucchinis, spiralized
- 2 tablespoons olive oil
- 1 cup coconut cream
- 2 cloves garlic, minced
- Salt and pepper to taste
- 1/4 cup grated Parmesan cheese (optional for non-dairy)
- Fresh parsley, chopped for garnish

Instructions:

1. Heat 1 tablespoon olive oil in a large skillet over medium heat. Add shrimp and cook until pink, about 2-3 minutes per side. Remove shrimp and set aside.
2. In the same skillet, add the remaining olive oil and garlic. Sauté for 1 minute until fragrant.
3. Add coconut cream and bring to a simmer. Reduce heat and let simmer for 5 minutes, until the sauce thickens slightly.
4. Stir in the spiralized zucchini (zoodles) and cook for 2-3 minutes, until zoodles are tender.
5. Return shrimp to the skillet, tossing to combine. Season with salt and pepper.
6. Serve topped with Parmesan and parsley.

Nutritional Info (per serving):

- Calories: ~350
- Protein: 25g
- Fat: 22g
- Carbohydrates: 10g
- Fiber: 2g

Serves: 4

Cooking Time: 20 minutes

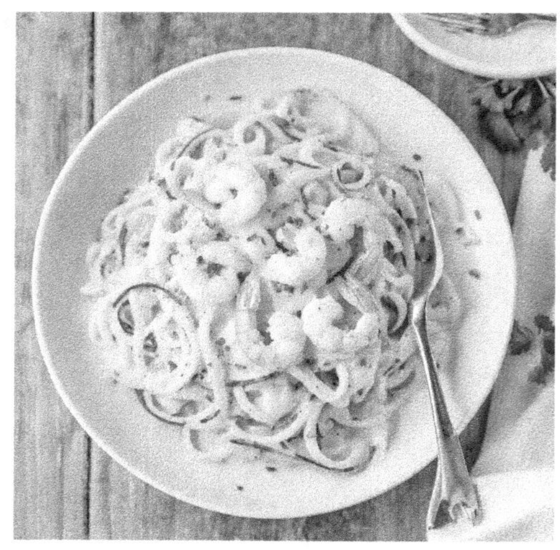

3. Thai Coconut Curry Mussels

Ingredients:

- 2 lbs fresh mussels, cleaned
- 1 can (14 oz) coconut milk
- 2 tablespoons red curry paste
- 1 tablespoon fish sauce
- 1 tablespoon brown sugar or coconut sugar
- 2 cloves garlic, minced
- 1 inch ginger, grated
- 1 red bell pepper, sliced
- 1/2 cup fresh basil leaves
- Lime wedges for serving

Instructions:

1. In a large pot, combine coconut milk, red curry paste, fish sauce, sugar, garlic, and ginger. Bring to a simmer over medium heat.
2. Add the mussels and red bell pepper to the pot. Cover and cook for 5-7 minutes, until mussels have opened. Discard any that do not open.
3. Stir in fresh basil just before serving.
4. Serve hot with lime wedges on the side.

Nutritional Info (per serving):

- Calories: ~300
- Protein: 22g
- Fat: 15g
- Carbohydrates: 15g
- Fiber: 1g

Serves: 4

Cooking Time: 15 minutes

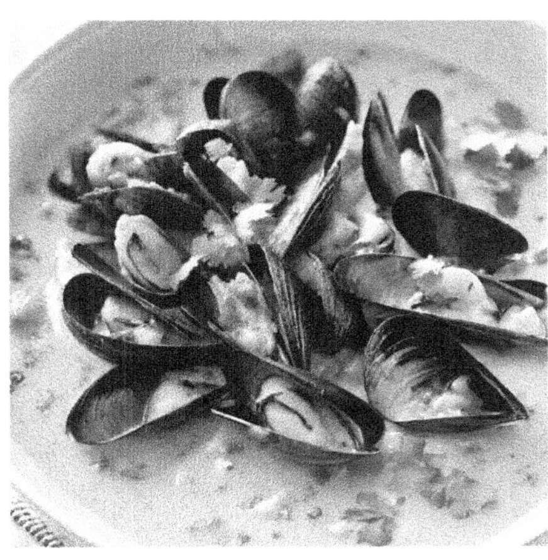

4. Moroccan Grilled Sardines

Ingredients:

- 2 lbs fresh sardines, cleaned
- 2 tablespoons olive oil
- 2 cloves garlic, minced
- 1 teaspoon paprika
- 1 teaspoon cumin
- Salt and pepper to taste
- Fresh lemon wedges for serving

Instructions:

1. In a small bowl, mix olive oil, garlic, paprika, cumin, salt, and pepper. Rub this mixture over the sardines.
2. Preheat the grill to medium-high heat. Grill sardines for 2-3 minutes per side, until cooked through and slightly charred.
3. Serve immediately with fresh lemon wedges.

Nutritional Info (per serving):

- Calories: ~250
- Protein: 25g
- Fat: 15g
- Carbohydrates: 1g
- Fiber: 0g

Serves: 4

Cooking Time: 10 minutes

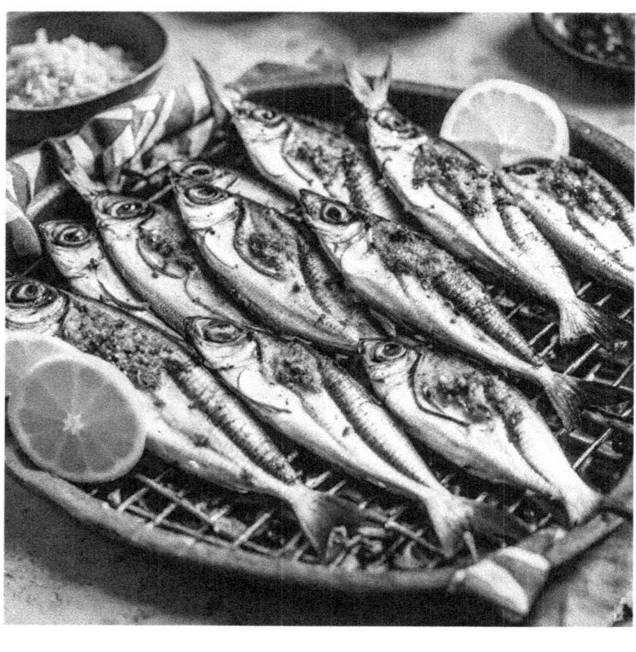

5. Baked Cod with Lemon and Dill

Ingredients:

- 4 cod fillets (about 6 oz each)
- 2 tablespoons olive oil
- Juice and zest of 1 lemon
- 2 cloves garlic, minced
- 2 tablespoons fresh dill, chopped
- Salt and pepper to taste
- Lemon slices for garnish

Instructions:

1. Preheat the oven to 400°F (200°C).
2. In a small bowl, combine olive oil, lemon juice and zest, garlic, dill, salt, and pepper.
3. Place cod fillets in a baking dish. Pour the lemon and dill mixture over the cod, ensuring each piece is well coated.
4. Bake in the preheated oven for 12-15 minutes, or until the cod is flaky and cooked through.
5. Garnish with lemon slices and additional fresh dill before serving.

Nutritional Info (per serving):

- Calories: ~200
- Protein: 30g
- Fat: 9g
- Carbohydrates: 2g
- Fiber: 0g

Serves: 4

Cooking Time: 15 minutes

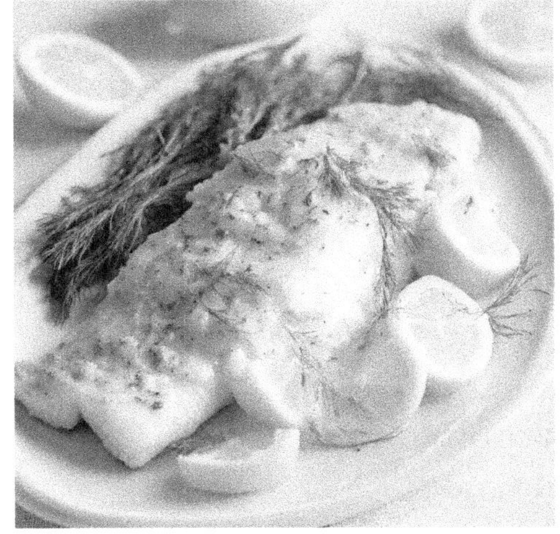

6. Paleo Paella

Ingredients:

- 2 tablespoons olive oil
- 1 lb chicken thighs, cut into pieces
- 1 lb shrimp, peeled and deveined
- 1 large onion, diced
- 1 red bell pepper, sliced
- 2 cloves garlic, minced
- 1 cup cauliflower rice
- 1 cup diced tomatoes
- 2 cups chicken broth
- 1 teaspoon saffron threads
- 1 teaspoon smoked paprika
- Salt and pepper to taste
- 1/2 cup fresh parsley, chopped
- Lemon wedges for serving

Instructions:

1. Heat olive oil in a large skillet over medium-high heat. Add chicken and cook until browned. Remove and set aside.
2. In the same skillet, add shrimp and cook until pink. Remove and set aside.
3. Sauté onion, bell pepper, and garlic until soft. Add cauliflower rice, diced tomatoes, chicken broth, saffron, and smoked paprika. Season with salt and pepper.
4. Return chicken to the skillet. Cover and simmer for 20 minutes.
5. Add shrimp back to the skillet, warming through.
6. Garnish with parsley and serve with lemon wedges.

Nutritional Info (per serving):

- Calories: ~300
- Protein: 35g
- Fat: 12g
- Carbohydrates: 12g
- Fiber: 3g

Serves: 4

Cooking Time: 40 minutes

7. Italian Seafood Stew

Ingredients:

- 1 tablespoon olive oil
- 1 onion, chopped
- 3 cloves garlic, minced
- 1 can (14 oz) diced tomatoes
- 1 cup fish or vegetable broth
- 1/2 cup white wine (optional)
- 1 lb mixed seafood (shrimp, scallops, calamari)
- 1 teaspoon dried basil
- 1 teaspoon dried oregano
- Salt and pepper to taste
- Fresh parsley for garnish

Instructions:

1. Heat olive oil in a large pot over medium heat. Add onion and garlic, cooking until soft.
2. Add diced tomatoes, broth, and white wine. Bring to a simmer.
3. Add seafood, basil, and oregano. Season with salt and pepper.
4. Cook until seafood is cooked through, about 5-7 minutes.
5. Garnish with fresh parsley before serving.

Nutritional Info (per serving):

- Calories: ~250
- Protein: 25g
- Fat: 8g
- Carbohydrates: 10g
- Fiber: 2g

Serves: 4

Cooking Time: 25 minutes

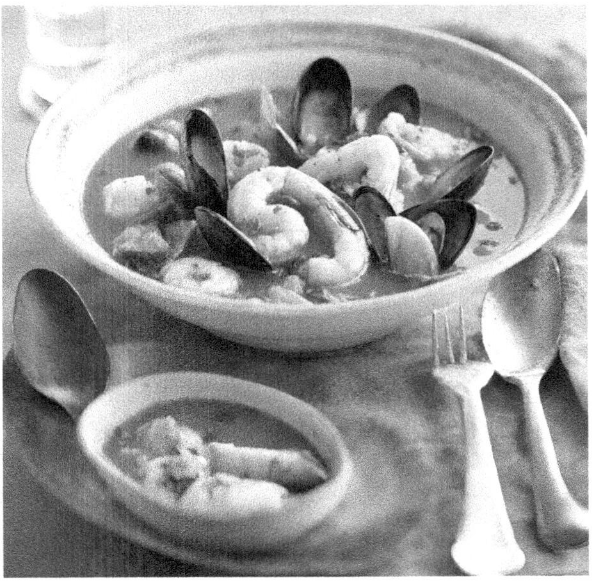

8. Salmon Poke Bowl

Ingredients:

- 1 lb fresh salmon, cubed
- 2 cups cooked cauliflower rice, cooled
- 1 avocado, sliced
- 1/2 cucumber, sliced
- 1 carrot, julienned
- 2 tablespoons soy sauce (gluten-free)
- 1 tablespoon sesame oil
- 1 teaspoon rice vinegar
- 1 teaspoon honey (optional)
- Sesame seeds for garnish
- Green onions, chopped for garnish

Instructions:

1. In a bowl, whisk together soy sauce, sesame oil, rice vinegar, and honey. Add salmon cubes and marinate for 10-15 minutes.
2. Divide cauliflower rice among bowls. Top with marinated salmon, avocado slices, cucumber, and carrot.
3. Garnish with sesame seeds and green onions.

Nutritional Info (per serving):

- Calories: ~350
- Protein: 25g
- Fat: 22g
- Carbohydrates: 12g
- Fiber: 4g

Serves: 4

Cooking Time: 20 minutes (excluding rice cooking time)

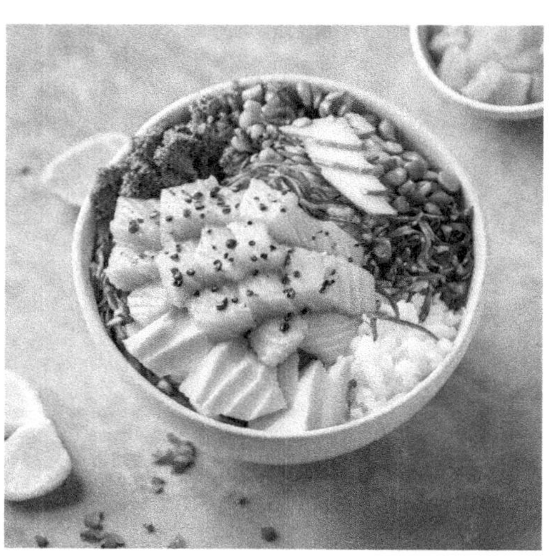

9. Garlic-Lime Shrimp

Ingredients:

- 1 lb shrimp, peeled and deveined
- 2 tablespoons olive oil
- 4 cloves garlic, minced
- Juice of 1 lime
- Zest of 1 lime
- Salt and pepper to taste
- Fresh parsley, chopped for garnish

Instructions:

1. Heat olive oil in a skillet over medium heat. Add garlic and cook until fragrant, about 1 minute.
2. Add shrimp, lime juice, and lime zest. Season with salt and pepper.
3. Cook until shrimp are pink and cooked through, about 3-5 minutes.
4. Garnish with parsley before serving.

Nutritional Info (per serving):

- Calories: ~180
- Protein: 24g
- Fat: 8g
- Carbohydrates: 3g
- Fiber: 0g

Serves: 4

Cooking Time: 10 minute

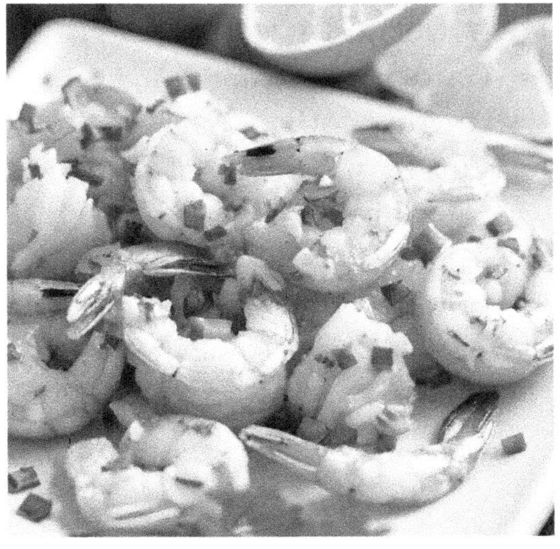

10. Bouillabaisse

Ingredients:

- 1 tablespoon olive oil
- 1 onion, chopped
- 2 cloves garlic, minced
- 1 fennel bulb, chopped
- 1 can (14 oz) diced tomatoes
- 4 cups fish or vegetable broth
- 1 pinch saffron threads
- 1 teaspoon thyme
- 1 bay leaf
- 1 lb mixed fish fillets (such as cod, halibut), cut into pieces
- 1 lb shellfish (such as shrimp, mussels, clams)
- Salt and pepper to taste
- Fresh parsley, chopped for garnish

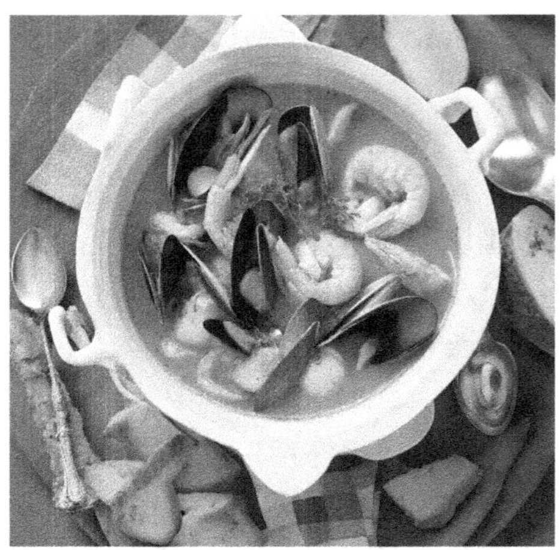

Instructions:

1. In a large pot, heat olive oil over medium heat. Add onion, garlic, and fennel, cooking until softened.
2. Stir in diced tomatoes, broth, saffron, thyme, and bay leaf. Bring to a simmer.
3. Add fish and shellfish. Season with salt and pepper. Cover and cook until fish is flaky and shellfish have opened, about 10-15 minutes.
4. Discard any unopened shellfish. Garnish with fresh parsley before serving.

Nutritional Info (per serving):

- Calories: ~300
- Protein: 40g
- Fat: 8g
- Carbohydrates: 15g
- Fiber: 3g

Serves: 4

Cooking Time: 30 minutes

11. Tandoori Prawns

Ingredients:

- 1 lb large prawns, peeled and deveined
- 1 cup plain yogurt (dairy-free if needed)
- 2 tablespoons tandoori masala
- 1 tablespoon lemon juice
- 1 teaspoon garlic, minced
- 1 teaspoon ginger, minced
- Salt to taste
- Fresh cilantro for garnish

Instructions:

1. In a bowl, mix together yogurt, tandoori masala, lemon juice, garlic, ginger, and salt. Add prawns and marinate for at least 1 hour, preferably overnight.
2. Preheat the grill to medium-high heat. Thread prawns onto skewers.
3. Grill for 2-3 minutes on each side, until cooked through and slightly charred.
4. Garnish with cilantro before serving.

Nutritional Info (per serving):

- Calories: ~200
- Protein: 24g
- Fat: 8g
- Carbohydrates: 5g
- Fiber: 0g

Serves: 4

Cooking Time: 10 minutes (excluding marinating time)

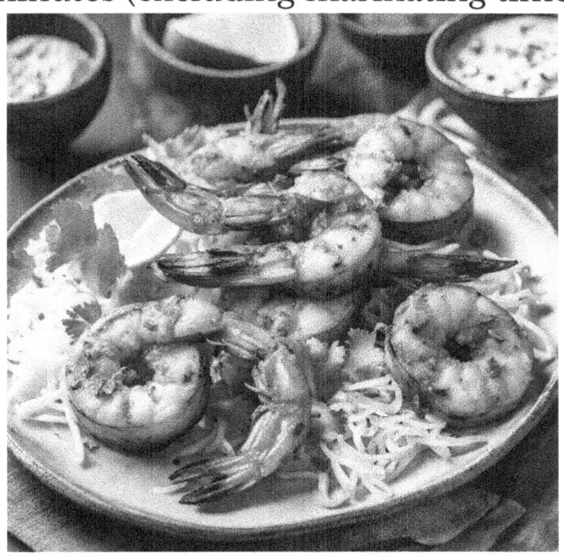

12. Smoked Salmon Breakfast Salad

Ingredients:

- 4 cups mixed greens
- 8 oz smoked salmon, sliced
- 1 avocado, sliced
- 4 poached eggs
- 1/4 cup capers
- 2 tablespoons olive oil
- 1 tablespoon lemon juice
- Salt and pepper to taste

Instructions:

1. Divide the mixed greens among four plates. Top each with smoked salmon, avocado slices, and a poached egg.
2. Sprinkle capers over each salad.
3. In a small bowl, whisk together olive oil, lemon juice, salt, and pepper. Drizzle over the salads.
4. Serve immediately.

Nutritional Info (per serving):

- Calories: ~300
- Protein: 23g
- Fat: 20g
- Carbohydrates: 8g
- Fiber: 4g

Serves: 4
Cooking Time: 20 minutes

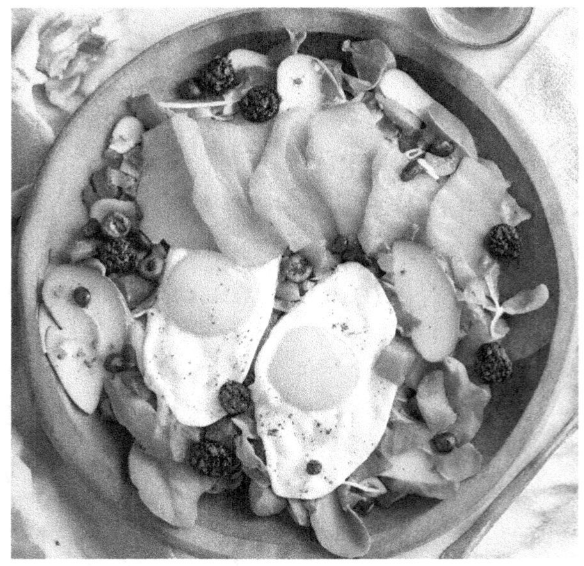

13. Prawn Tikka

Ingredients:

- 1 lb large prawns, peeled and deveined
- 1 cup plain yogurt (dairy-free if needed)
- 2 tablespoons tikka masala paste
- 1 tablespoon lemon juice
- Salt to taste
- Fresh cilantro and lemon wedges for serving

Instructions:

1. In a bowl, combine yogurt, tikka masala paste, lemon juice, and salt. Add prawns and marinate for at least 1 hour, up to overnight.
2. Preheat the grill to medium-high heat. Thread marinated prawns onto skewers.
3. Grill for 2-3 minutes on each side, until prawns are pink and slightly charred.
4. Serve garnished with cilantro and lemon wedges.

Nutritional Info (per serving):

- Calories: ~200
- Protein: 25g
- Fat: 8g
- Carbohydrates: 5g
- Fiber: 0g

Serves: 4

Cooking Time: 10 minutes (excluding marinating time)

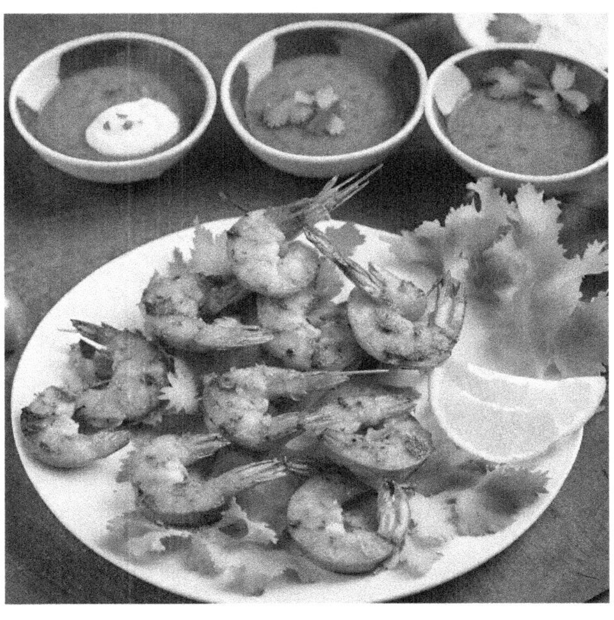

14. Lemon Dill Scallop Skewers

Ingredients:

- 1 lb large scallops
- 2 tablespoons olive oil
- Juice and zest of 1 lemon
- 2 tablespoons fresh dill, chopped
- Salt and pepper to taste
- Wooden skewers, soaked in water

Instructions:

1. In a bowl, mix olive oil, lemon juice and zest, dill, salt, and pepper. Add scallops and marinate for 30 minutes.
2. Thread scallops onto soaked skewers.
3. Preheat grill to medium-high heat. Grill skewers for 2-3 minutes per side, until scallops are opaque and slightly charred.
4. Serve immediately.

Nutritional Info (per serving):

- Calories: ~200
- Protein: 20g
- Fat: 10g
- Carbohydrates: 5g
- Fiber: 0g

Serves: 4

Cooking Time: 6 minutes (excluding marinating time)

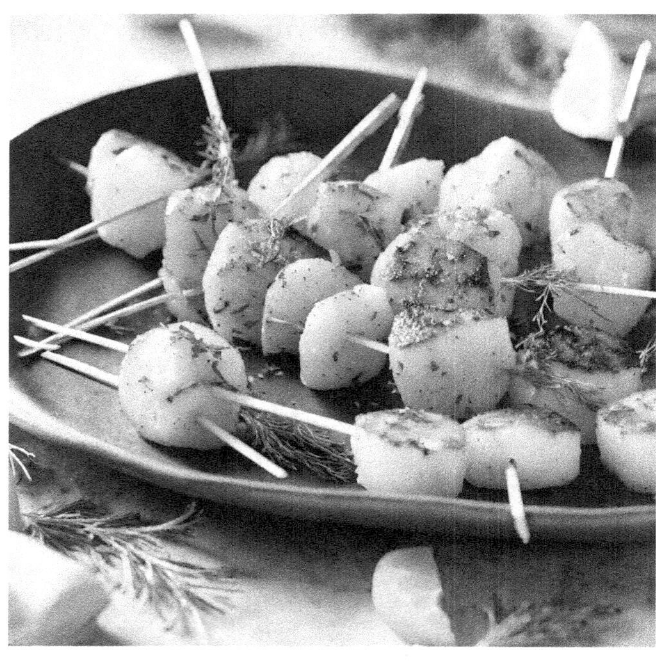

15. Halibut Piccata

Ingredients:

- 4 halibut fillets (6 oz each)
- 2 tablespoons olive oil
- 1/4 cup flour (for dusting, optional)
- 2 cloves garlic, minced
- Juice of 1 lemon
- 1/4 cup capers, drained
- 1/2 cup vegetable broth
- Salt and pepper to taste
- Fresh parsley, chopped for garnish

Instructions:

1. Season halibut with salt and pepper. Lightly dust with flour if desired.
2. Heat olive oil in a skillet over medium heat. Add halibut and cook until golden brown, about 3-4 minutes per side. Remove and set aside.
3. In the same skillet, add garlic, lemon juice, capers, and broth. Simmer until the sauce reduces slightly.
4. Return halibut to the skillet, warming through.
5. Garnish with parsley before serving.

Nutritional Info (per serving):

- Calories: ~300
- Protein: 35g
- Fat: 15g
- Carbohydrates: 5g
- Fiber: 0g

Serves: 4

Cooking Time: 20 minutes

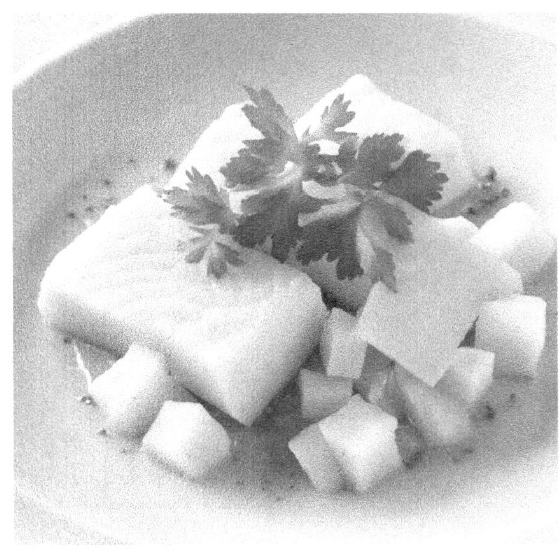

16. Cajun Catfish

Ingredients:

- 4 catfish fillets (6 oz each)
- 2 tablespoons Cajun seasoning
- 2 tablespoons olive oil
- Lemon wedges for serving

Instructions:

1. Rub Cajun seasoning all over the catfish fillets.
2. Heat olive oil in a skillet over medium heat. Add catfish and cook for 4-5 minutes per side, until crispy and cooked through.
3. Serve with lemon wedges.

Nutritional Info (per serving):

- Calories: ~250
- Protein: 22g
- Fat: 16g
- Carbohydrates: 1g
- Fiber: 0g

Serves: 4

Cooking Time: 10 minutes

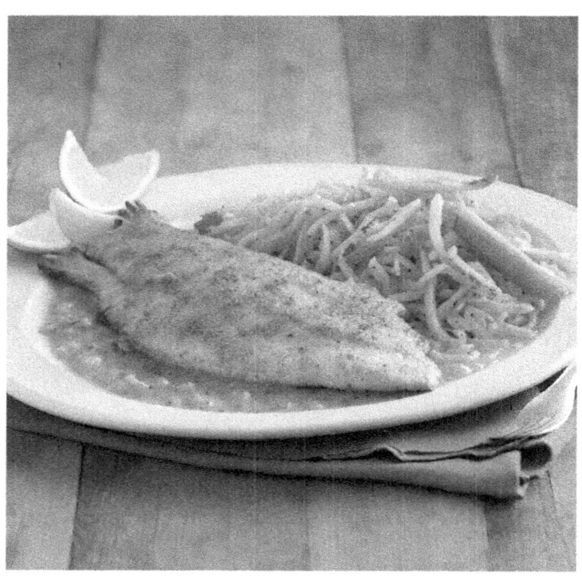

17. Greek Grilled Octopus

Ingredients:

- 1 lb octopus, cleaned
- 2 tablespoons olive oil
- 2 cloves garlic, minced
- Juice of 1 lemon
- 1 tablespoon oregano
- Salt and pepper to taste
- Lemon wedges for serving

Instructions:

1. Pre-cook octopus in boiling water for 40-60 minutes until tender. Cool and cut into pieces.
2. Marinate octopus in olive oil, garlic, lemon juice, oregano, salt, and pepper for at least 1 hour.
3. Preheat grill to medium-high. Grill octopus pieces until charred, about 2-3 minutes per side.
4. Serve with lemon wedges.

Nutritional Info (per serving):

- Calories: ~200
- Protein: 25g
- Fat: 10g
- Carbohydrates: 5g
- Fiber: 0g

Serves: 4

Cooking Time: 1 hour 10 minutes (including pre-cooking and marinating)

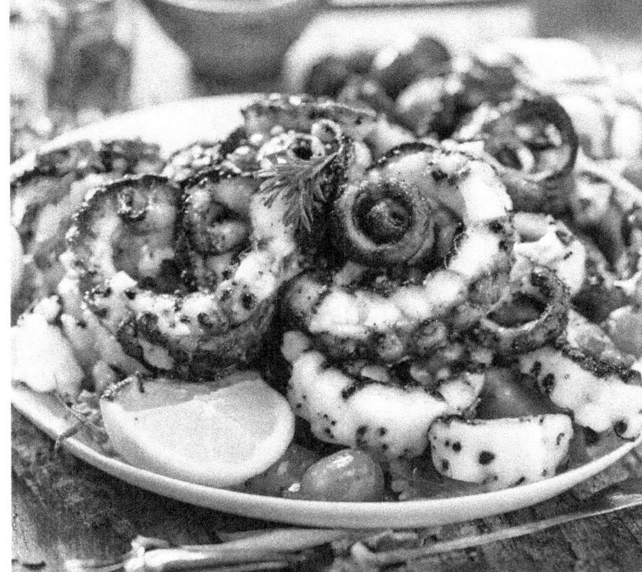

18. Brazilian Moqueca

Ingredients:

- 1 lb firm white fish (e.g., cod, halibut), cut into chunks
- 1 lb shrimp, peeled and deveined
- 2 tablespoons lime juice
- 2 tablespoons olive oil
- 1 onion, sliced
- 1 red bell pepper, sliced
- 2 cloves garlic, minced
- 1 can (14 oz) coconut milk
- 1 can (14 oz) diced tomatoes
- 1 tablespoon paprika
- 1 tablespoon cilantro, chopped
- Salt and pepper to taste

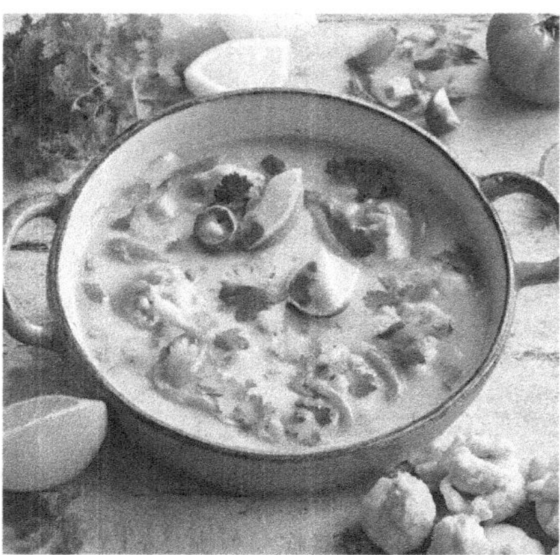

Instructions:

1. Marinate fish and shrimp in lime juice, salt, and pepper for 30 minutes.
2. Heat olive oil in a large pot over medium heat. Sauté onion, bell pepper, and garlic until soft.
3. Add coconut milk, diced tomatoes, and paprika. Bring to a simmer.
4. Add the marinated fish and shrimp to the pot. Cover and simmer gently for about 15-20 minutes, until the seafood is cooked through.
5. Garnish with chopped cilantro before serving.

Nutritional Info (per serving):

- Calories: ~350
- Protein: 35g
- Fat: 18g
- Carbohydrates: 12g
- Fiber: 3g

Serves: 4

Cooking Time: 50 minutes (including marinating time)

19. Baked Lemon Sole with Capers

Ingredients:

- 4 sole fillets (about 6 oz each)
- 2 tablespoons olive oil
- Juice and zest of 1 lemon
- 2 tablespoons capers, drained
- Salt and pepper to taste
- Fresh parsley, chopped for garnish

Instructions:

1. Preheat the oven to 375°F (190°C).
2. Place sole fillets in a baking dish. Drizzle with olive oil and lemon juice. Sprinkle lemon zest and capers over the top. Season with salt and pepper.
3. Bake for 12-15 minutes, until the fish flakes easily with a fork.
4. Garnish with fresh parsley before serving.

Nutritional Info (per serving):

- Calories: ~200
- Protein: 23g
- Fat: 10g
- Carbohydrates: 2g
- Fiber: 0g

Serves: 4

Cooking Time: 15 minutes

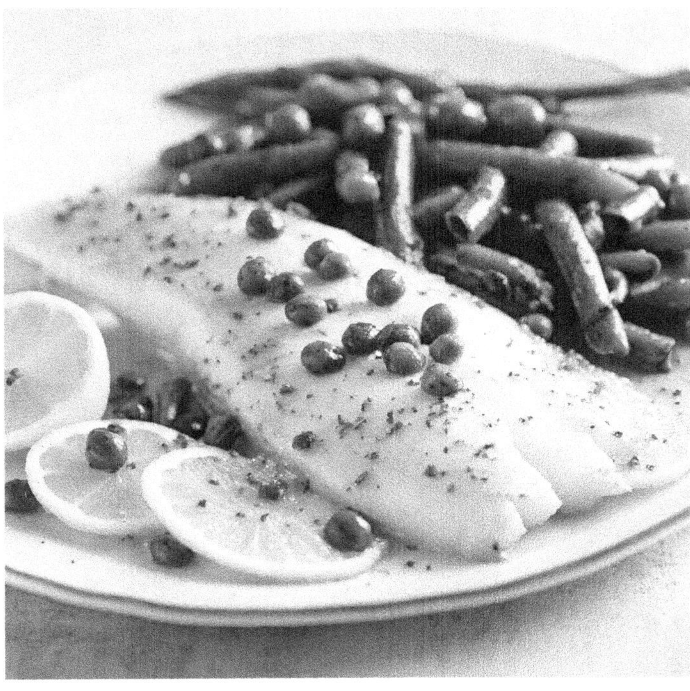

20. Crab Salad with Citrus Vinaigrette

Ingredients:

- 1 lb crab meat, cooked and shredded
- 4 cups mixed greens
- 1 avocado, sliced
- 1 orange, segmented
- 1/4 cup sliced almonds
- For the vinaigrette:
  - 1/4 cup olive oil
  - Juice of 1 lemon
  - Juice of 1 orange
  - 1 teaspoon honey
  - Salt and pepper to taste

Instructions:

1. In a large bowl, combine crab meat, mixed greens, avocado slices, and orange segments.
2. In a small bowl, whisk together all vinaigrette ingredients until well combined.
3. Pour the vinaigrette over the salad and toss gently to coat.
4. Sprinkle sliced almonds on top before serving.

Nutritional Info (per serving):

- Calories: ~300
- Protein: 20g
- Fat: 20g
- Carbohydrates: 12g
- Fiber: 5g

Serves: 4

Cooking Time: 15 minutes

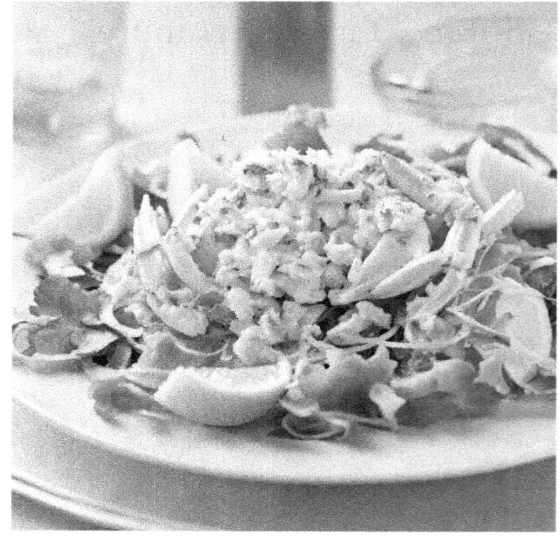

21. Korean Grilled Mackerel

Ingredients:

- 2 whole mackerel, gutted and cleaned
- 2 tablespoons soy sauce (gluten-free)
- 1 tablespoon sesame oil
- 1 tablespoon garlic, minced
- 1 tablespoon ginger, minced
- 1 tablespoon gochugaru (Korean red pepper flakes)
- 1 tablespoon honey
- Salt to taste
- Sliced green onions and sesame seeds for garnish

Instructions:

1. Score the mackerel on both sides. Mix soy sauce, sesame oil, garlic, ginger, gochugaru, honey, and salt in a bowl to make the marinade.
2. Rub the marinade all over the mackerel, inside and out. Let marinate for at least 30 minutes.
3. Preheat the grill to medium-high heat. Grill the mackerel for 4-5 minutes on each side, until the skin is crisp and the fish is cooked through.
4. Garnish with sliced green onions and sesame seeds before serving.

Nutritional Info (per serving):

- Calories: ~350
- Protein: 23g
- Fat: 25g
- Carbohydrates: 8g
- Fiber: 1g

Serves: 4

Cooking Time: 40 minutes (including marinating time)

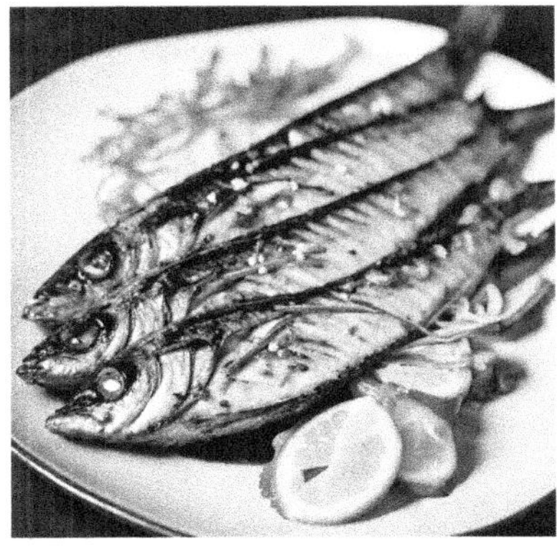

VEGETABLES AND SALAD

1. Roasted Cauliflower Steak

Ingredients:

- 1 large head cauliflower
- 2 tablespoons olive oil
- 1 teaspoon garlic powder
- 1 teaspoon paprika
- Salt and pepper to taste

Instructions:

1. Preheat the oven to 400°F (200°C).
2. Slice the cauliflower head into 1-inch thick steaks, ensuring the core keeps each steak intact.
3. Mix olive oil, garlic powder, paprika, salt, and pepper in a bowl. Brush this mixture on both sides of each cauliflower steak.
4. Place cauliflower steaks on a baking sheet lined with parchment paper.
5. Roast in the oven for 25-30 minutes, flipping halfway through, until tender and golden.

Nutritional Info (per serving):

- Calories: ~110 Protein: 4g Fat: 7g
- Carbohydrates: 10g
- Fiber: 4g

Serves: 4

Cooking Time: 30 minutes

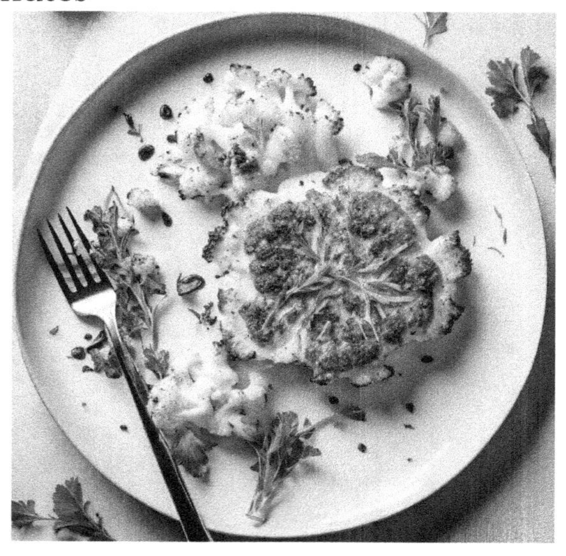

2. Kale and Brussels Sprout Salad

Ingredients:

- 2 cups kale, thinly sliced
- 2 cups Brussels sprouts, thinly sliced
- 1/4 cup almonds, chopped
- 1/4 cup Parmesan cheese, grated (optional)
- 2 tablespoons olive oil
- 1 tablespoon lemon juice
- 1 teaspoon Dijon mustard
- Salt and pepper to taste

Instructions:

1. In a large bowl, combine kale and Brussels sprouts.
2. In a small bowl, whisk together olive oil, lemon juice, Dijon mustard, salt, and pepper to create the dressing.
3. Pour the dressing over the kale and Brussels sprouts, tossing well to coat.
4. Add almonds and Parmesan cheese, and toss again.
5. Let the salad sit for about 10 minutes before serving to allow the kale to soften.

Nutritional Info (per serving):

- Calories: ~150 Protein: 5g Fat: 12g Carbohydrates: 8g
- Fiber: 3g

Serves: 4

Cooking Time: 15 minutes

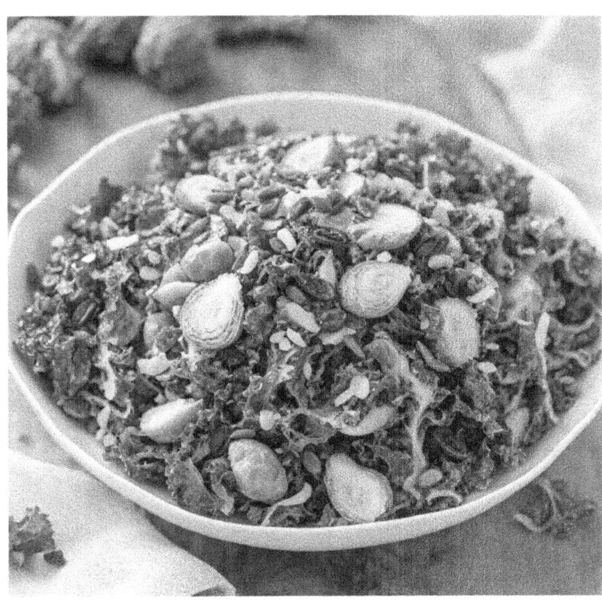

3. Spicy Roasted Sweet Potatoes

Ingredients:

- 2 large sweet potatoes, peeled and cubed
- 2 tablespoons olive oil
- 1 teaspoon chili powder
- 1/2 teaspoon cumin
- 1/2 teaspoon paprika
- Salt and pepper to taste

Instructions:

1. Preheat the oven to 425°F (220°C).
2. In a large bowl, toss sweet potatoes with olive oil, chili powder, cumin, paprika, salt, and pepper until well coated.
3. Spread the sweet potatoes in a single layer on a baking sheet lined with parchment paper.
4. Roast for 25-30 minutes, stirring halfway through, until tender and lightly caramelized.

Nutritional Info (per serving):

- Calories: ~200
- Protein: 2g
- Fat: 7g
- Carbohydrates: 34g
- Fiber: 5g

Serves: 4

Cooking Time: 30 minutes

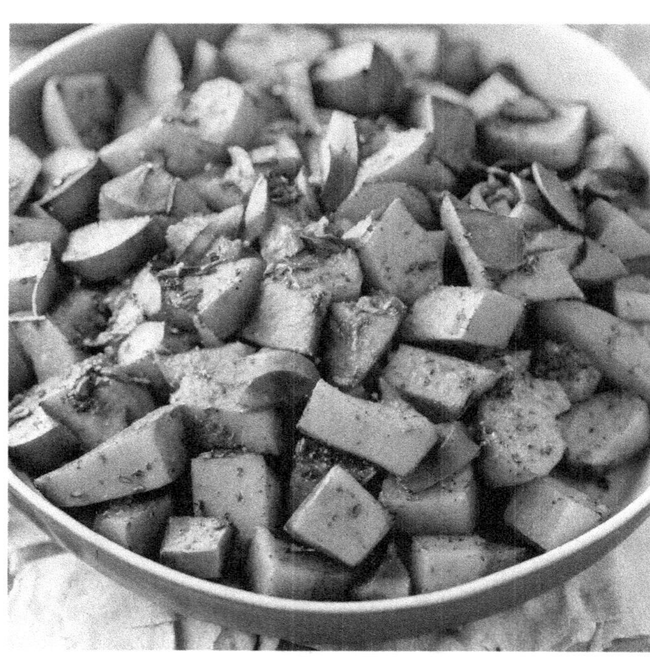

4. Quinoa Tabbouleh

Ingredients:

- 1 cup quinoa, cooked and cooled
- 1 cup parsley, finely chopped
- 1/2 cup mint, finely chopped
- 2 tomatoes, diced
- 1 cucumber, diced
- 1/4 cup lemon juice
- 2 tablespoons olive oil
- Salt and pepper to taste

Instructions:

1. In a large bowl, mix the cooked quinoa, parsley, mint, tomatoes, and cucumber.
2. In a small bowl, whisk together lemon juice, olive oil, salt, and pepper to create the dressing.
3. Pour the dressing over the quinoa mixture and toss well to combine.
4. Chill in the refrigerator for at least 30 minutes before serving to allow flavors to meld.

Nutritional Info (per serving):

- Calories: ~22G Protein: 6g Fat: 10g
- Carbohydrates: 30g
- Fiber: 5g

Serves: 4

Cooking Time: 40 minutes (including cooling time)

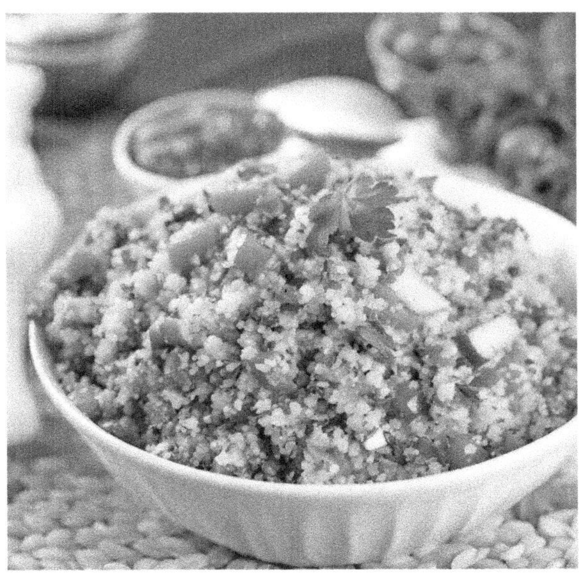

5. Balsamic Grilled Vegetables

Ingredients:

- 1 zucchini, sliced
- 1 yellow squash, sliced
- 1 red bell pepper, sliced
- 1 red onion, sliced
- 2 tablespoons olive oil
- 2 tablespoons balsamic vinegar
- Salt and pepper to taste

Instructions:

1. Preheat the grill to medium-high heat.
2. In a large bowl, toss the vegetables with olive oil, balsamic vinegar, salt, and pepper until well coated.
3. Place the vegetables on the grill, or use a grill basket to prevent them from falling through the grates.
4. Grill for 10-15 minutes, turning occasionally, until the vegetables are tender and have nice grill marks.
5. Serve immediately, optionally drizzling with a bit more balsamic vinegar before serving.

Nutritional Info (per serving):

- Calories: ~120
- Protein: 2g
- Fat: 7g
- Carbohydrates: 13g
- Fiber: 3g

Serves: 4

Cooking Time: 15 minutes

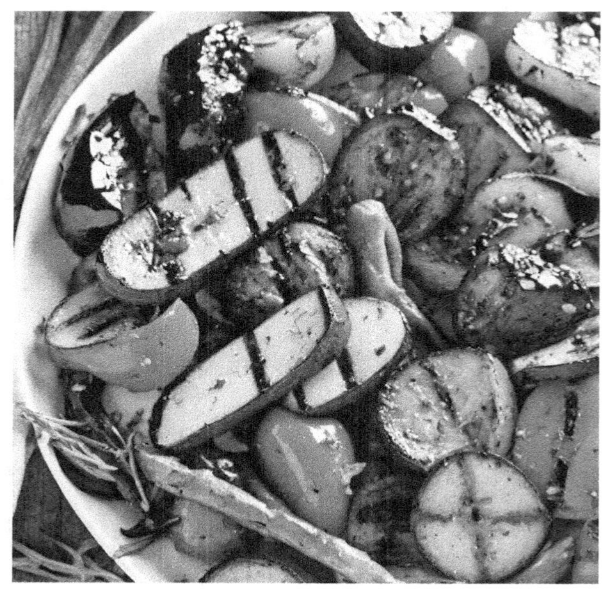

6. Asian Cucumber Salad

Ingredients:

- 2 large cucumbers, thinly sliced
- 1/4 cup rice vinegar
- 1 tablespoon sesame oil
- 1 tablespoon soy sauce (gluten-free)
- 1 teaspoon honey or sugar
- 1 clove garlic, minced
- 1 teaspoon sesame seeds
- 1/4 teaspoon red pepper flakes (optional)
- Salt to taste
- Fresh cilantro or green onions for garnish

Instructions:

1. In a large bowl, combine the cucumbers with a pinch of salt. Let sit for 10 minutes, then drain any excess liquid.
2. In a small bowl, whisk together rice vinegar, sesame oil, soy sauce, honey, garlic, sesame seeds, and red pepper flakes.
3. Pour the dressing over the cucumbers and toss to coat evenly.
4. Garnish with fresh cilantro or green onions before serving. Best served chilled.

Nutritional Info (per serving):

- Calories: ~70
- Protein: 1g
- Fat: 4g
- Carbohydrates: 8g
- Fiber: 1g

Serves: 4

Cooking Time: 20 minutes (including resting time)

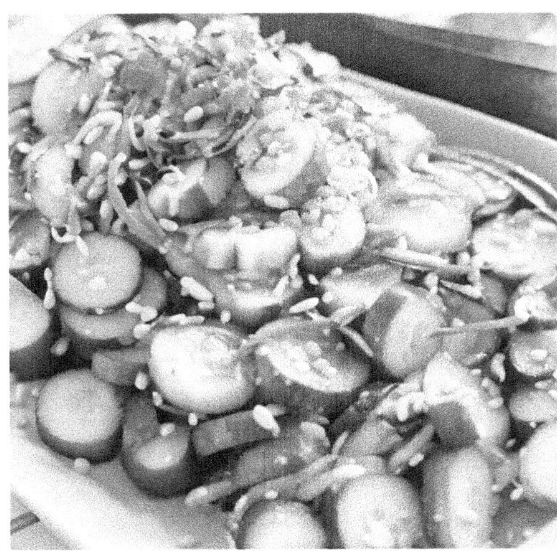

7. Eggplant Caponata

Ingredients:

- 2 large eggplants, cubed
- 3 tablespoons olive oil
- 1 onion, diced
- 2 cloves garlic, minced
- 1 red bell pepper, diced
- 1 can (14 oz) diced tomatoes
- 3 tablespoons capers, drained
- 2 tablespoons red wine vinegar
- 1 tablespoon sugar or honey
- Salt and pepper to taste
- Fresh basil for garnish

Instructions:

1. Preheat the oven to 375°F (190°C). Toss eggplant cubes with 2 tablespoons olive oil and spread on a baking sheet. Roast for 25-30 minutes until tender.
2. In a large pan, heat the remaining olive oil over medium heat. Add onion, garlic, and bell pepper, cooking until softened.
3. Stir in roasted eggplant, diced tomatoes, capers, vinegar, and sugar. Simmer for 15 minutes. Season with salt and pepper.
4. Garnish with fresh basil before serving. Can be served warm or cold.

Nutritional Info (per serving):

- Calories: ~180
- Protein: 3g
- Fat: 7g
- Carbohydrates: 28g
- Fiber: 9g

Serves: 4

Cooking Time: 45 minutes

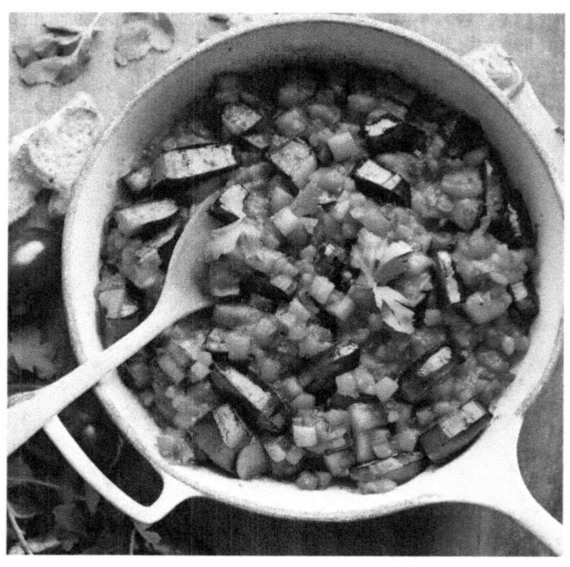

8. Greek Salad

Ingredients:

- 3 tomatoes, chopped
- 1 cucumber, sliced
- 1 red onion, thinly sliced
- 1/2 cup Kalamata olives
- 1/2 cup feta cheese, crumbled (optional for dairy-free)
- 3 tablespoons olive oil
- 1 tablespoon red wine vinegar
- 1 teaspoon dried oregano
- Salt and pepper to taste

Instructions:

1. In a large bowl, combine tomatoes, cucumber, red onion, olives, and feta cheese.
2. In a small bowl, whisk together olive oil, red wine vinegar, oregano, salt, and pepper.
3. Pour dressing over the salad and gently toss to combine.
4. Serve immediately or let chill in the refrigerator for 30 minutes to enhance flavors.

Nutritional Info (per serving):

- Calories: ~200
- Protein: 4g
- Fat: 16g
- Carbohydrates: 10g
- Fiber: 2g

Serves: 4

Cooking Time: 10 minutes

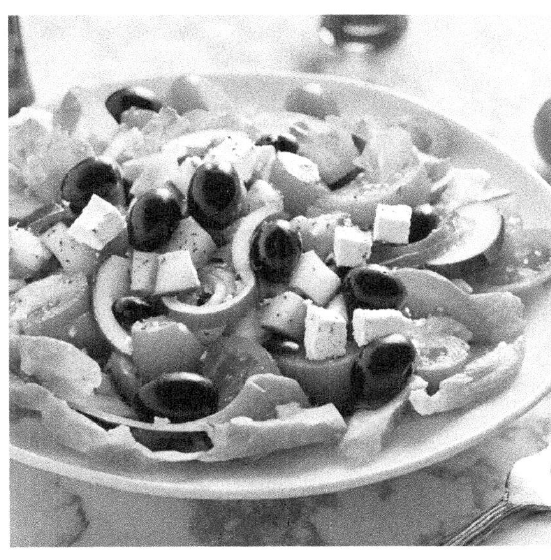

9. Mexican Street Corn Salad

Ingredients:

- 4 cups corn kernels (fresh, frozen, or canned)
- 1 tablespoon olive oil
- 1/2 cup mayonnaise or Greek yogurt (dairy-free if needed)
- 1 lime, juiced
- 1 teaspoon chili powder
- 1/4 cup fresh cilantro, chopped
- 1/4 cup cotija cheese or feta (optional for dairy-free)
- Salt and pepper to taste

Instructions:

1. Heat olive oil in a large skillet over medium heat. Add corn and cook until charred, about 10 minutes.
2. Remove from heat and let cool slightly. Transfer to a large bowl.
3. Stir in mayonnaise, lime juice, chili powder, cilantro, and cheese. Season with salt and pepper.
4. Serve warm or at room temperature.

Nutritional Info (per serving):

- Calories: ~250
- Protein: 5g
- Fat: 16g
- Carbohydrates: 24g
- Fiber: 3g

Serves: 4
Cooking Time: 15 minutes

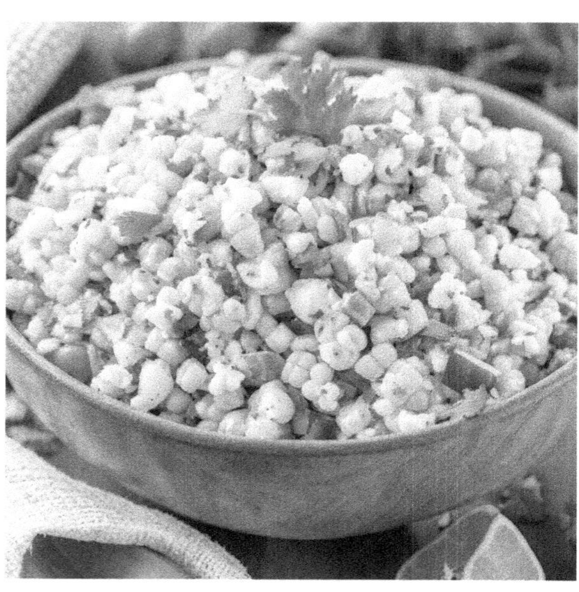

10. Spinach and Strawberry Salad

Ingredients:

- 4 cups fresh spinach leaves
- 1 cup strawberries, sliced
- 1/2 cup walnuts, toasted
- 1/4 cup balsamic vinegar
- 2 tablespoons olive oil
- 1 tablespoon honey (optional)
- Salt and pepper to taste
- 1/4 cup goat cheese, crumbled (optional for dairy-free)

Instructions:

1. In a large bowl, combine spinach, strawberries, and walnuts.
2. In a small bowl, whisk together balsamic vinegar, olive oil, honey, salt, and pepper to create the dressing.
3. Pour dressing over the salad and toss gently to combine.
4. Top with crumbled goat cheese, if using, before serving.

Nutritional Info (per serving):

- Calories: ~220
- Protein: 6g
- Fat: 18g
- Carbohydrates: 12g
- Fiber: 3g

Serves: 4

Cooking Time: 10 minutes

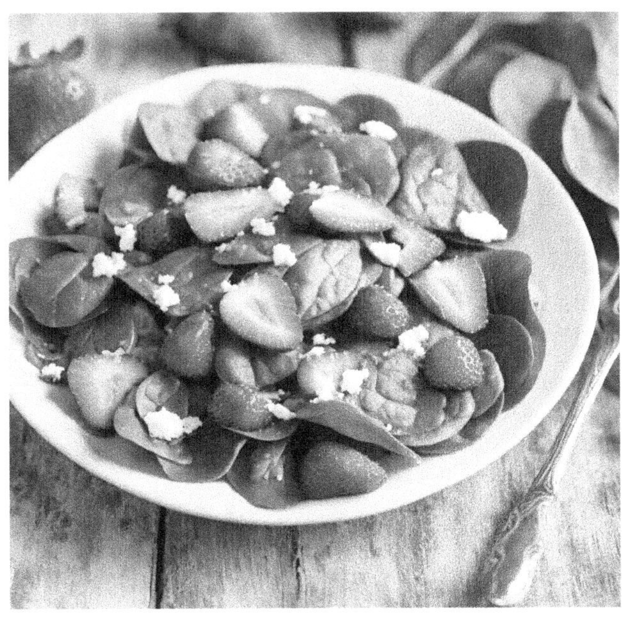

11. Butternut Squash Risotto

Ingredients:

- 1 medium butternut squash, peeled and cubed
- 2 tablespoons olive oil, divided
- 1 small onion, finely chopped
- 2 cloves garlic, minced
- 1 cup arborio rice
- 1/2 cup white wine (optional)
- 4 cups vegetable broth, warmed
- Salt and pepper to taste
- 1/4 cup grated Parmesan cheese (optional for dairy-free)
- Fresh sage for garnish

Instructions:

1. Preheat the oven to 400°F (200°C). Toss butternut squash cubes with 1 tablespoon olive oil, salt, and pepper. Roast for 25-30 minutes until tender.
2. In a large pan, heat the remaining olive oil over medium heat. Add onion and garlic, sautéing until soft.
3. Stir in arborio rice, toasting for 1-2 minutes. Add white wine, stirring until absorbed.
4. Add warmed vegetable broth 1/2 cup at a time, stirring frequently, until each addition is absorbed before adding more.
5. Once the rice is cooked and creamy, stir in roasted butternut squash. Season with salt and pepper.
6. Serve garnished with Parmesan cheese and fresh sage.

Nutritional Info (per serving):

- Calories: ~350
- Protein: 8g
- Fat: 9g
- Carbohydrates: 60g
- Fiber: 4g

Serves: 4

Cooking Time: 1 hour

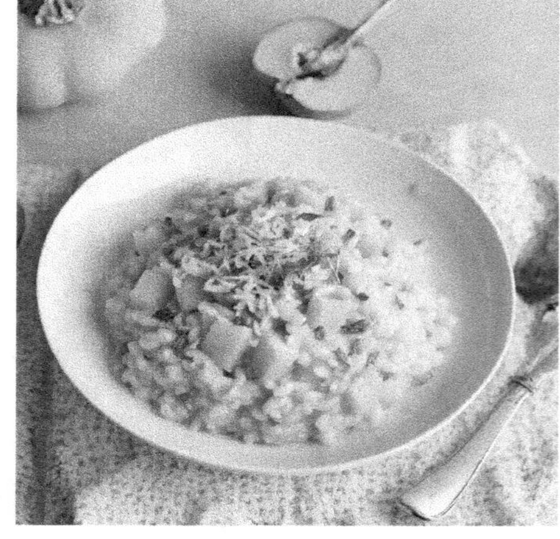

12. Avocado Tomato Salad

Ingredients:

- 2 ripe avocados, diced
- 2 large tomatoes, diced
- 1/4 cup red onion, finely chopped
- 2 tablespoons olive oil
- 1 tablespoon lime juice
- Salt and pepper to taste
- Fresh cilantro for garnish

Instructions:

1. In a large bowl, combine avocados, tomatoes, and red onion.
2. Drizzle with olive oil and lime juice, then season with salt and pepper.
3. Toss gently to combine.
4. Garnish with fresh cilantro before serving.

Nutritional Info (per serving):

- Calories: ~220
- Protein: 3g
- Fat: 20g
- Carbohydrates: 12g
- Fiber: 7g

Serves: 4

Cooking Time: 10 minutes

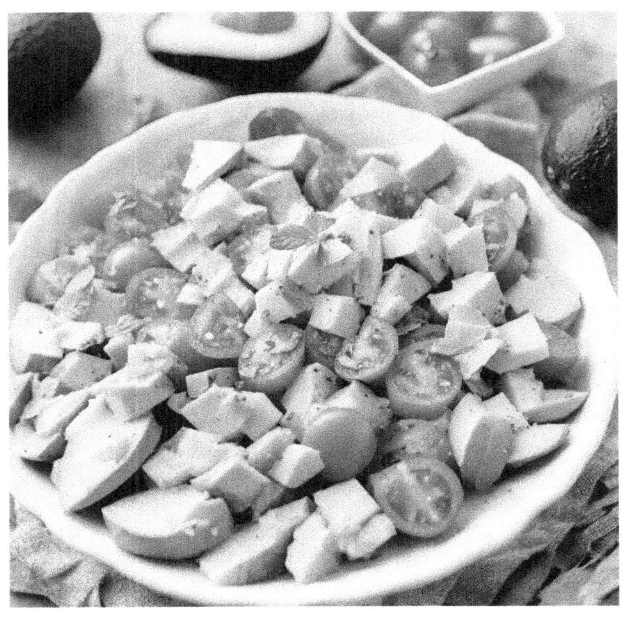

13. Zucchini Ribbon Salad

Ingredients:

- 2 large zucchinis
- 2 tablespoons olive oil
- 1 tablespoon lemon juice
- Salt and pepper to taste
- 1/4 cup shaved Parmesan cheese (optional for dairy-free)
- Pine nuts for garnish

Instructions:

1. Use a vegetable peeler or mandoline to slice zucchinis into thin ribbons.
2. In a large bowl, whisk together olive oil, lemon juice, salt, and pepper.
3. Add zucchini ribbons to the dressing, tossing gently to coat.
4. Top with shaved Parmesan and pine nuts before serving.

Nutritional Info (per serving):

- Calories: ~120
- Protein: 4g
- Fat: 10g
- Carbohydrates: 4g
- Fiber: 1g

Serves: 4
Cooking Time: 15 minutes

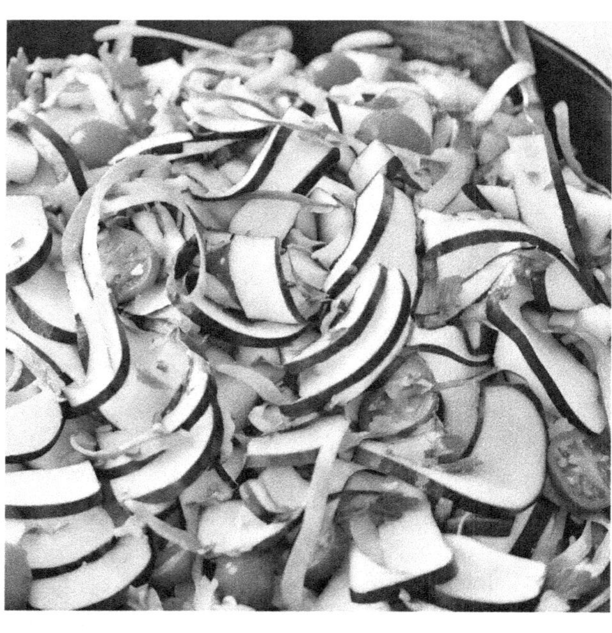

14. Warm Mushroom Salad

Ingredients:

- 4 cups mixed mushrooms, sliced (e.g., shiitake, button, portobello)
- 2 tablespoons olive oil
- 2 cloves garlic, minced
- 4 cups mixed greens (e.g., arugula, spinach)
- 1 tablespoon balsamic vinegar
- Salt and pepper to taste
- Shaved Parmesan cheese (optional for dairy-free)

Instructions:

1. In a large skillet, heat olive oil over medium heat. Add mushrooms and garlic, sautéing until mushrooms are tender and browned.
2. Toss the warm mushrooms with mixed greens and balsamic vinegar. Season with salt and pepper.
3. Serve immediately, topped with shaved Parmesan if desired.

Nutritional Info (per serving):

- Calories: ~110
- Protein: 3g
- Fat: 7g
- Carbohydrates: 10g
- Fiber: 2g

Serves: 4

Cooking Time: 20 minutes

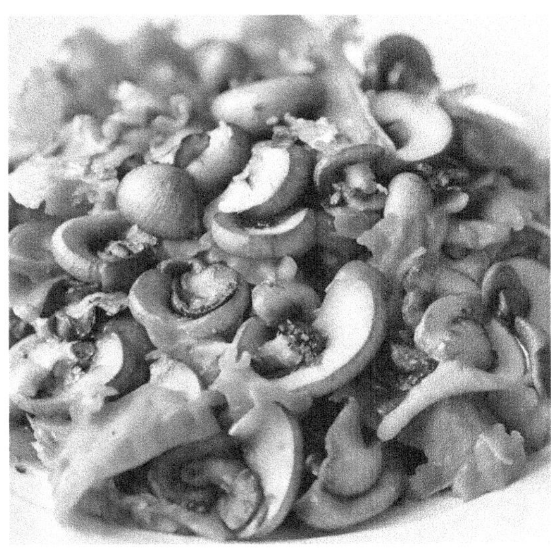

15. Broccoli and Apple Salad
Ingredients:
- 4 cups broccoli florets, chopped
- 1 large apple, diced
- 1/2 cup red onion, finely chopped
- 1/2 cup walnuts, chopped
- 1/2 cup dried cranberries
- 1/4 cup mayonnaise (use a vegan version for dairy-free)
- 2 tablespoons apple cider vinegar
- 1 tablespoon honey (or a vegan alternative)
- Salt and pepper to taste

Instructions:
1. In a large bowl, combine broccoli, apple, red onion, walnuts, and dried cranberries.
2. In a small bowl, whisk together mayonnaise, apple cider vinegar, and honey. Season with salt and pepper.
3. Pour the dressing over the broccoli mixture and toss to coat evenly.
4. Chill in the refrigerator for at least 30 minutes before serving to allow flavors to meld.

Nutritional Info (per serving):
- Calories: ~250
- Protein: 4g
- Fat: 15g
- Carbohydrates: 28g
- Fiber: 4g

Serves: 4
Cooking Time: 10 minutes (plus chilling time)

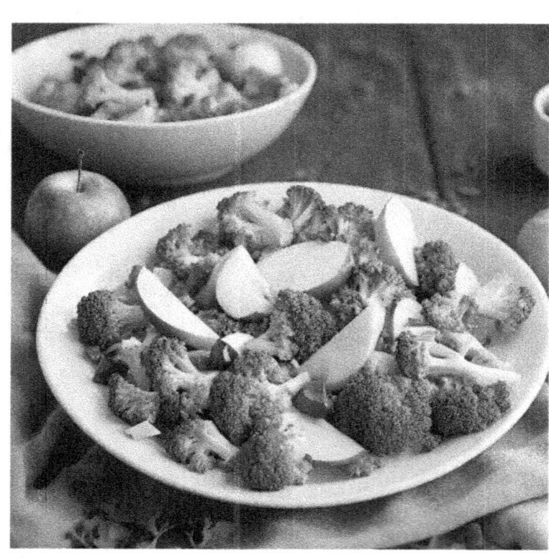

16. Sweet Potato and Black Bean Salad
Ingredients:

- 2 large sweet potatoes, peeled and cubed
- 1 tablespoon olive oil
- 1 can (15 oz) black beans, drained and rinsed
- 1 red bell pepper, diced
- 1/2 red onion, finely chopped
- 1/4 cup fresh cilantro, chopped
- Juice of 1 lime
- 1 teaspoon chili powder
- Salt and pepper to taste

Instructions:

1. Preheat the oven to 400°F (200°C). Toss sweet potatoes with olive oil, salt, and pepper. Spread on a baking sheet and roast for 25 minutes, until tender.
2. In a large bowl, combine roasted sweet potatoes, black beans, red bell pepper, red onion, and cilantro.
3. Add lime juice and chili powder, tossing to coat. Season with salt and pepper to taste.
4. Serve warm or at room temperature.

Nutritional Info (per serving):

- Calories: ~220 Protein: 7g Fat: 4g
- Carbohydrates: 40g
- Fiber: 10g

Serves: 4
Cooking Time: 35 minutes

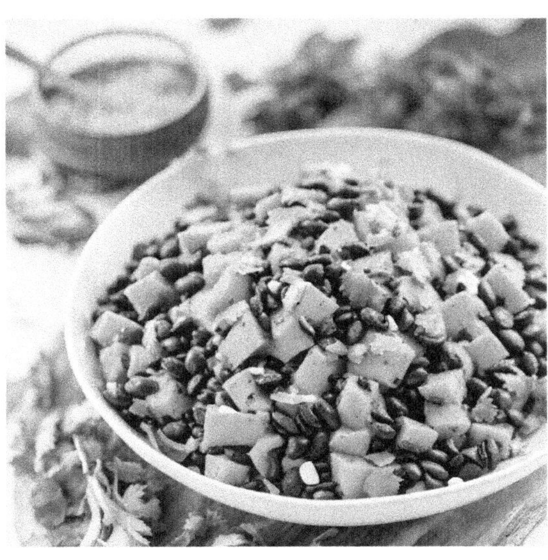

17. Mediterranean Lentil Salad

Ingredients:

- 2 cups cooked lentils
- 1 cucumber, diced
- 1 tomato, diced
- 1/2 red onion, finely chopped
- 1/4 cup olives, sliced
- 1/4 cup feta cheese, crumbled (optional for dairy-free)
- 3 tablespoons olive oil
- 2 tablespoons red wine vinegar
- 1 teaspoon dried oregano
- Salt and pepper to taste

Instructions:

1. In a large bowl, combine lentils, cucumber, tomato, red onion, olives, and feta cheese.
2. In a small bowl, whisk together olive oil, red wine vinegar, oregano, salt, and pepper.
3. Pour the dressing over the lentil mixture and toss to coat evenly.
4. Chill for at least 1 hour before serving to allow flavors to develop.

Nutritional Info (per serving):

- Calories: ~300 Protein: 14g Fat: 14g
- Carbohydrates: 34g
- Fiber: 12g

Serves: 4

Cooking Time: 15 minutes (plus chilling time)

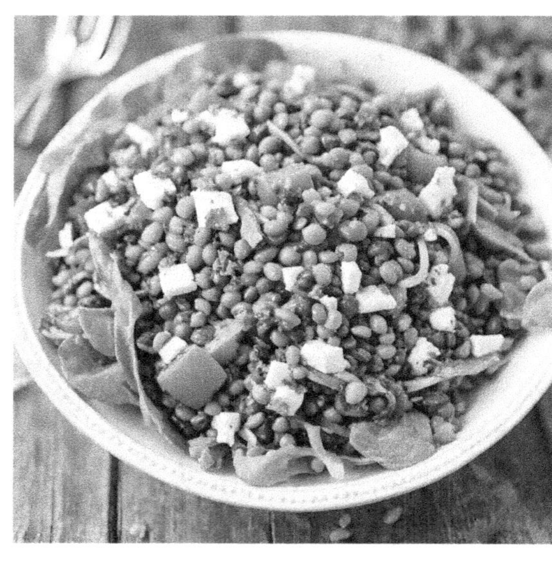

18. Cucumber Gazpacho

Ingredients:

- 2 large cucumbers, peeled and chopped
- 1 green bell pepper, chopped
- 1 small onion, chopped
- 2 cloves garlic, minced
- 2 cups vegetable broth, chilled
- 1/4 cup fresh parsley, chopped
- 2 tablespoons lime juice
- Salt and pepper to taste
- 1/4 cup Greek yogurt (optional for dairy-free, can use coconut yogurt)

Instructions:

1. In a blender, combine cucumbers, bell pepper, onion, garlic, vegetable broth, parsley, and lime juice. Blend until smooth.
2. Season with salt and pepper to taste.
3. Chill for at least 2 hours before serving.
4. Serve garnished with a dollop of Greek yogurt if desired.

Nutritional Info (per serving):

- Calories: ~70
- Protein: 3g
- Fat: 0.5g
- Carbohydrates: 15g
- Fiber: 2g

Serves: 4

Cooking Time: 10 minutes (plus at least 2 hours chilling)

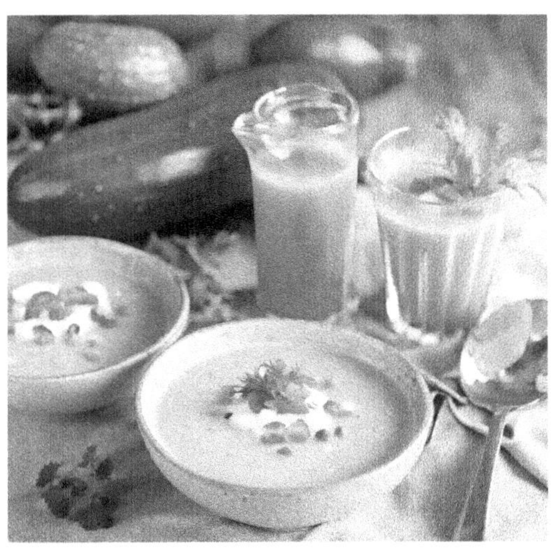

19. Roasted Brussels Sprouts with Pomegranate

Ingredients:

- 1 lb Brussels sprouts, halved
- 2 tablespoons olive oil
- Salt and pepper to taste
- 1/2 cup pomegranate seeds
- 2 tablespoons balsamic glaze

Instructions:

1. Preheat the oven to 400°F (200°C).
2. Toss Brussels sprouts with olive oil, salt, and pepper on a baking sheet.
3. Roast for 20-25 minutes until crispy on the outside and tender on the inside.
4. Transfer to a serving dish and sprinkle with pomegranate seeds.
5. Drizzle with balsamic glaze before serving.

Nutritional Info (per serving):

- Calories: ~150
- Protein: 4g
- Fat: 7g
- Carbohydrates: 20g
- Fiber: 5g

Serves: 4

Cooking Time: 25 minutes

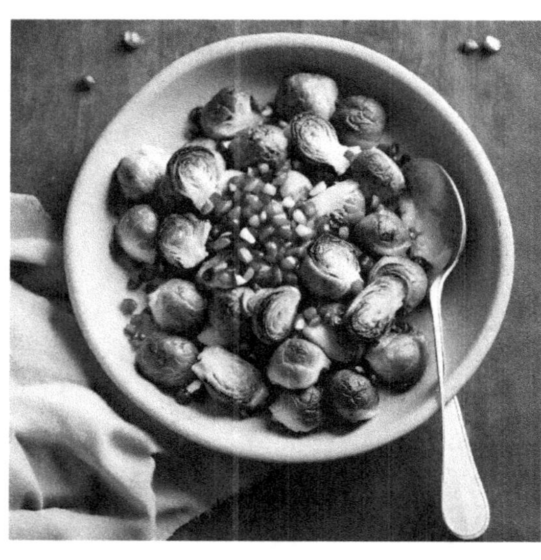

20. Thai Peanut Zucchini Noodles

Ingredients:

- 4 medium zucchinis, spiralized
- 1 carrot, julienned
- 1 red bell pepper, thinly sliced
- 1/4 cup creamy peanut butter
- 2 tablespoons soy sauce (gluten-free)
- 1 tablespoon lime juice
- 1 tablespoon honey or maple syrup
- 1 clove garlic, minced
- 1 teaspoon ginger, grated
- 1/4 cup cilantro, chopped
- 2 tablespoons peanuts, chopped for garnish

Instructions:

1. In a large bowl, combine zucchini noodles, carrot, and red bell pepper.
2. In a small bowl, whisk together peanut butter, soy sauce, lime juice, honey, garlic, and ginger until smooth.
3. Pour the peanut sauce over the zucchini noodle mixture and toss to coat evenly.
4. Garnish with cilantro and chopped peanuts before serving.

Nutritional Info (per serving):

- Calories: ~220 Protein: 8g Fat: 14g
- Carbohydrates: 18g
- Fiber: 4g

Serves: 4

Cooking Time: 15 minutes

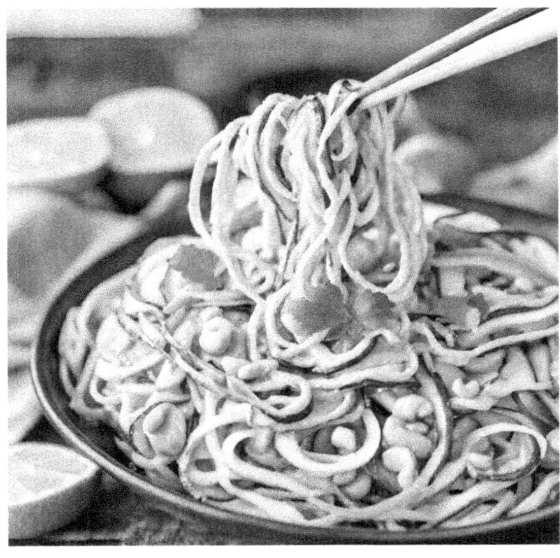

21. Sautéed Green Beans with Garlic

Ingredients:

- 1 lb green beans, trimmed
- 2 tablespoons olive oil
- 3 cloves garlic, minced
- Salt and pepper to taste
- Lemon wedges for serving

Instructions:

1. Heat olive oil in a large skillet over medium heat.
2. Add green beans and cook, stirring occasionally, until they start to soften, about 5 minutes.
3. Add minced garlic and continue to sauté for another 2-3 minutes until garlic is fragrant and beans are tender.
4. Season with salt and pepper.
5. Serve with lemon wedges.

Nutritional Info (per serving):

- Calories: ~90
- Protein: 2g
- Fat: 7g
- Carbohydrates: 8g
- Fiber: 3g

Serves: 4

Cooking Time: 10 minutes

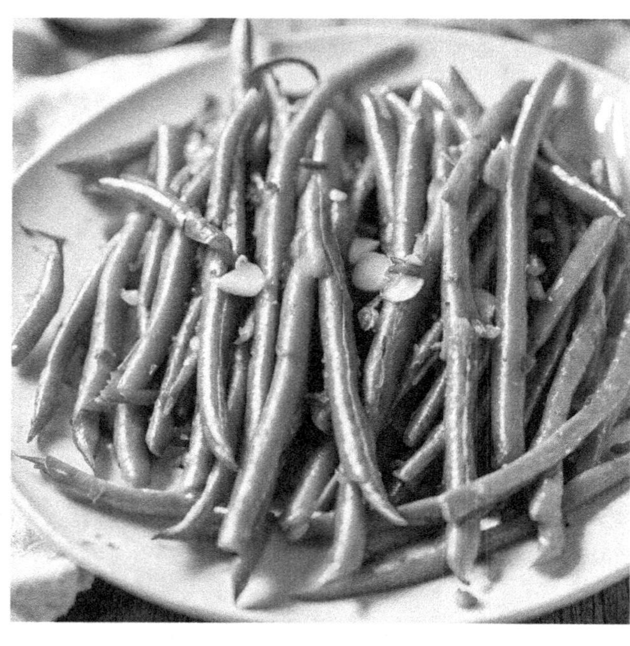

22. Watermelon and Feta Salad

Ingredients:

- 4 cups watermelon, cubed
- 1/2 cup feta cheese, crumbled (optional for dairy-free)
- 1/4 cup fresh mint, chopped
- 2 tablespoons olive oil
- 1 tablespoon balsamic vinegar
- Salt and pepper to taste

Instructions:

1. In a large bowl, combine watermelon cubes, feta cheese, and fresh mint.
2. Drizzle with olive oil and balsamic vinegar. Gently toss to combine.
3. Season with salt and pepper to taste.
4. Serve chilled for best flavor.

Nutritional Info (per serving):

- Calories: ~160
- Protein: 4g
- Fat: 9g
- Carbohydrates: 18g
- Fiber: 1g

Serves: 4

Cooking Time: 10 minutes

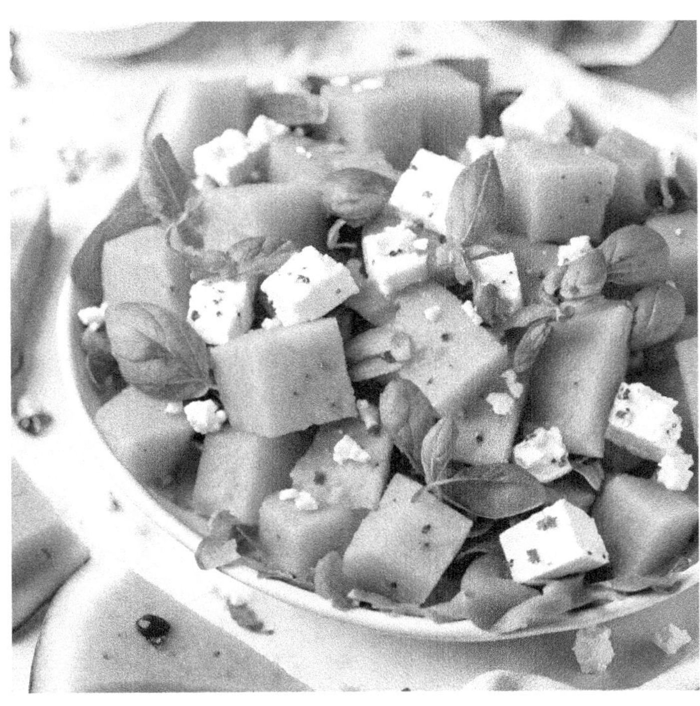

Moroccan Carrot Salad
Ingredients:
- 1 lb carrots, peeled and grated
- 1/4 cup olive oil
- 2 tablespoons lemon juice
- 2 cloves garlic, minced
- 1 teaspoon cumin
- 1/2 teaspoon cinnamon
- 1/4 teaspoon cayenne pepper (adjust according to taste)
- Salt to taste
- 1/4 cup chopped fresh parsley
- 2 tablespoons chopped fresh mint (optional)

Instructions:
1. In a large mixing bowl, combine the grated carrots with the chopped parsley and mint (if using).
2. In a small bowl, whisk together the olive oil, lemon juice, minced garlic, cumin, cinnamon, cayenne pepper, and salt until well combined.
3. Pour the dressing over the carrot mixture and toss until all the carrots are evenly coated with the dressing.
4. Cover and refrigerate for at least 30 minutes to allow the flavors to meld. This salad can be served chilled or at room temperature.
5. Before serving, give the salad a quick toss and adjust the seasoning if necessary.

Nutritional Info (per serving):
- Calories: ~150 Protein: 1g Fat: 10g
- Carbohydrates: 15g
- Fiber: 4g
- Sugar: 7g (natural sugars from carrots)

Serves: 4
Cooking Time: 10 minutes preparation, 30 minutes chilling

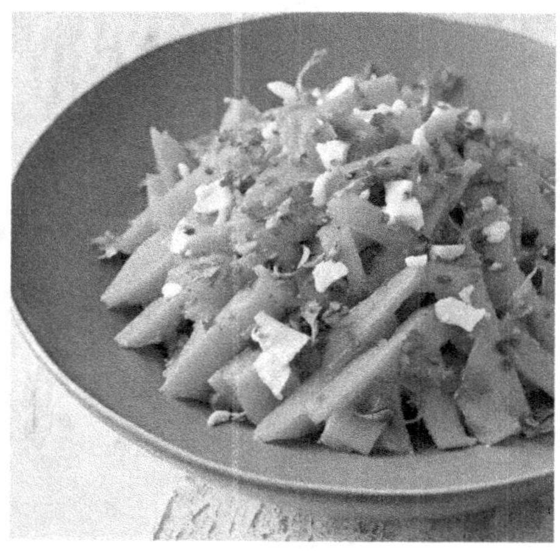

7-WEEK MEAL PLAN

Week 1

Monday
- Breakfast: Gluten-Free Oatmeal
- Lunch: Greek Salad
- Dinner: Grilled Salmon with Avocado Salsa

Tuesday
- Breakfast: Banana Almond Butter Smoothie
- Lunch: Sweet Potato and Black Bean Salad
- Dinner: Thai Coconut Curry Mussels

Wednesday
- Breakfast: Paleo Banana Bread
- Lunch: Avocado Tomato Salad
- Dinner: Italian Seafood Stew

Thursday
- Breakfast: Quinoa Porridge
- Lunch: Kale and Brussels Sprout Salad
- Dinner: Ethiopian Doro Wat

Friday
- Breakfast: Coconut Yogurt Parfait
- Lunch: Spinach and Strawberry Salad
- Dinner: Moroccan Grilled Sardines

Saturday
- Breakfast: Smoked Salmon Breakfast Salad
- Lunch: Butternut Squash Risotto
- Dinner: Mexican Street Corn Salad with Grilled Chicken

Sunday
- Breakfast: Egg Muffins
- Lunch: Zucchini Ribbon Salad
- Dinner: Bouillabaisse

Week 2

Monday
- Breakfast: Baked Eggs in Avocado
- Lunch: Moroccan Carrot Salad
- Dinner: Cajun Catfish

Tuesday
- Breakfast: Pumpkin Seed Oatmeal
- Lunch: Mediterranean Lentil Salad
- Dinner: Paleo Paella

Wednesday
- Breakfast: Lemon Dill Scallop Skewers
- Lunch: Broccoli and Apple Salad
- Dinner: Lemon Dill Scallop Skewers

Thursday
- Breakfast: Paleo Breakfast Muffins
- Lunch: Asian Cucumber Salad
- Dinner: Roasted Brussels Sprouts with Pomegranate

Friday
- Breakfast: Banana Almond Butter Smoothie (repeat)
- Lunch: Watermelon and Feta Salad
- Dinner: Greek Grilled Octopus

Saturday
- Breakfast: Quinoa Porridge (repeat)
- Lunch: Sautéed Green Beans with Garlic
- Dinner: Thai Peanut Zucchini Noodles

Sunday
- Breakfast: Coconut Yogurt Parfait (repeat)
- Lunch: Eggplant Caponata
- Dinner: Brazilian Moqueca

Week 3
Monday
- Breakfast: Gluten-Free Oatmeal (repeat)
- Lunch: Cucumber Gazpacho
- Dinner: Halibut Piccata

Tuesday

- Breakfast: Smoothie of choice (Banana Almond Butter or another)
- Lunch: Quinoa Tabbouleh
- Dinner: Sweet Potato and Black Bean Salad (repeat)

Wednesday

- Breakfast: Egg Muffins (repeat)
- Lunch: Greek Salad (repeat)
- Dinner: Tandoori Prawns

Thursday

- Breakfast: Paleo Banana Bread (repeat)
- Lunch: Warm Mushroom Salad
- Dinner: Salmon Poke Bowl

Friday

- Breakfast: Baked Eggs in Avocado (repeat)
- Lunch: Zucchini Ribbon Salad (repeat)
- Dinner: Spicy Roasted Sweet Potatoes

Saturday

- Breakfast: Quinoa Porridge (repeat)
- Lunch: Broccoli and Apple Salad (repeat)
- Dinner: Korean Grilled Mackerel

Sunday

- Breakfast: Smoothie of choice
- Lunch: Moroccan Carrot Salad (repeat)
- Dinner: Italian Seafood Stew (repeat)

Week 4

Monday

- Breakfast: Chia Seed Pudding with Fresh Berries
- Lunch: Roasted Beet and Goat Cheese Salad
- Dinner: Grilled Lemon-Garlic Shrimp Skewers

Tuesday

- Breakfast: Dairy-Free Frittata with Spinach and Mushrooms
- Lunch: Quinoa and Black Bean Stuffed Peppers
- Dinner: Beef Stir-Fry with Broccoli and Bell Peppers

Wednesday
- Breakfast: Almond Flour Pancakes with Blueberry Sauce
- Lunch: Carrot Ginger Soup
- Dinner: Baked Tilapia with Dill and Mustard

Thursday
- Breakfast: Sweet Potato Hash with Poached Eggs
- Lunch: Avocado and Chicken Lettuce Wraps
- Dinner: Ratatouille with Grilled Chicken Breast

Friday
- Breakfast: Green Smoothie with Spinach, Avocado, and Pineapple
- Lunch: Lentil Soup with Leafy Greens
- Dinner: Seared Scallops with Cauliflower Puree

Saturday
- Breakfast: Paleo Granola with Coconut Yogurt
- Lunch: Tomato Basil Soup
- Dinner: Cod in Tomato and Olive Sauce

Sunday
- Breakfast: Poached Eggs with Avocado Toast (gluten-free bread)
- Lunch: Stuffed Avocados with Tuna Salad
- Dinner: Rosemary Lemon Chicken Thighs with Asparagus

Week 5
Monday
- Breakfast: Berry and Flaxseed Smoothie
- Lunch: Eggplant and Chickpea Stew
- Dinner: Turkey Meatballs in Tomato Basil Sauce

Tuesday
- Breakfast: Coconut Flour Waffles
- Lunch: Cucumber and Seaweed Salad
- Dinner: Pan-Seared Salmon with Walnut-Parsley Pesto

Wednesday
- Breakfast: Pumpkin Spice Smoothie
- Lunch: Roasted Red Pepper and Tomato Soup
- Dinner: Lemon Herb Roasted Chicken with Zucchini

Thursday
- Breakfast: Omelet with Spinach, Tomatoes, and Onions
- Lunch: Tuna Salad over Mixed Greens
- Dinner: Spaghetti Squash with Pesto and Cherry Tomatoes

Friday
- Breakfast: Apple Cinnamon Oatmeal (gluten-free oats)
- Lunch: Cold Lentil Salad with Cucumbers and Olives
- Dinner: Garlic Butter Baked Cod

Saturday
- Breakfast: Avocado and Berry Salad with Lemon Dressing
- Lunch: Quinoa Salad with Roasted Vegetables
- Dinner: Stir-Fried Tofu with Mixed Vegetables

Sunday
- Breakfast: Veggie-Packed Frittata
- Lunch: Chicken Avocado Salad
- Dinner: Baked Eggplant Parmesan (with gluten-free breadcrumbs)

Week 6
Monday
- Breakfast: Mango and Spinach Smoothie
- Lunch: Broccoli Salad with Bacon Bits
- Dinner: Grilled Trout with Lemon and Herbs

Tuesday
- Breakfast: Paleo Apple Muffins
- Lunch: Mediterranean Chickpea Salad
- Dinner: Pork Tenderloin with Roasted Apples and Onions

Wednesday
- Breakfast: Sweet Potato and Almond Butter Smoothie
- Lunch: Kale Caesar Salad (dairy-free dressing)
- Dinner: Chicken Curry with Coconut Milk

Thursday
- Breakfast: Banana Nut Porridge (gluten-free oats)
- Lunch: Sardine Salad on Mixed Greens
- Dinner: Vegetarian Chili

Friday
- Breakfast: Fruit Salad with Chia Seeds and Coconut Shavings
- Lunch: Beet and Walnut Salad
- Dinner: Shrimp and Asparagus Stir Fry

Saturday
- Breakfast: Paleo Blueberry Muffins
- Lunch: Chicken Soup with Vegetables
- Dinner: Grilled Lamb Chops with Mint Sauce

Sunday
- Breakfast: Veggie Hash with Eggs
- Lunch: Roasted Pumpkin Salad
- Dinner: Orange-Glazed Salmon with Steamed Broccoli

Week 7

Monday
- Breakfast: Kiwi and Spinach Smoothie
- Lunch: Cold Quinoa Salad with Lemon and Dill
- Dinner: Moroccan Spiced Chicken with Vegetable Couscous (gluten-free couscous)

Tuesday
- Breakfast: Gluten-Free Toast with Avocado and Radish
- Lunch: Zucchini Boats Filled with Ground Turkey and Tomato Sauce
- Dinner: Pan-Fried Haddock with Lemon Butter Sauce

Wednesday
- Breakfast: Raspberry Almond Smoothie Bowl
- Lunch: Arugula Salad with Grilled Peaches and Balsamic Glaze
- Dinner: Ginger-Soy Glazed Cod with Stir-Fried Vegetables

Thursday
- Breakfast: Overnight Chia Pudding with Almond Milk and Berries
- Lunch: Spinach and Quinoa Salad with Lemon Vinaigrette
- Dinner: Herb-Crusted Pork Chops with Roasted Sweet Potatoes

Friday
- Breakfast: Avocado Smoothie with Spinach and Coconut Water
- Lunch: Greek Chickpea Salad with Olives and Feta
- Dinner: Garlic and Rosemary Grilled Eggplant with Quinoa

Saturday
- Breakfast: Paleo Pancakes with Fresh Strawberry Compote
- Lunch: Cabbage and Carrot Slaw with Vinegar Dressing
- Dinner: Baked Lemon and Herb Salmon with Asparagus

FOOD TRACKER
JOURNAL

Dates

Shopping List

Foods to Avoid

	BREAKFAST	LUNCH	DINNER
MON			
TUE			
WED			
THU			
FRI			
SAT			
SUN			

Reflect on your current dietary habits. What are some common foods you consume on a daily basis?

Have you noticed any specific symptoms related to Hashimoto's Thyroiditis that you believe might be influenced by your diet?

What are your expectations and goals regarding the gluten-free diet in managing your Hashimoto's Thyroiditis?

FOOD TRACKER JOURNAL

	BREAKFAST	LUNCH	DINNER
MON			
TUE			
WED			
THU			
FRI			
SAT			
SUN			

Dates
____

Shopping List

Foods to Avoid

Describe any challenges or concerns you anticipate facing while transitioning to a gluten-free lifestyle.

What are your favorite gluten-containing foods, and how do you plan to replace or adapt them in your new diet?

FOOD TRACKER JOURNAL

	BREAKFAST	LUNCH	DINNER
MON			
TUE			
WED			
THU			
FRI			
SAT			
SUN			

Dates
____

Shopping List

Foods to Avoid

Reflect on potential barriers to adherence to the gluten-free diet, such as dining out or traveling. What strategies can you implement to overcome these challenges?

Imagine yourself six months from now. How do you envision your lifestyle and dietary habits having changed since starting the gluten-free diet?

FOOD TRACKER JOURNAL

Dates
____

Shopping List

	BREAKFAST	LUNCH	DINNER
MON			
TUE			
WED			
THU			
FRI			
SAT			
SUN			

Foods to Avoid

FOOD TRACKER JOURNAL

	BREAKFAST	LUNCH	DINNER
MON			
TUE			
WED			
THU			
FRI			
SAT			
SUN			

Dates
____

Shopping List

Foods to Avoid

FOOD TRACKER JOURNAL

	BREAKFAST	LUNCH	DINNER
MON			
TUE			
WED			
THU			
FRI			
SAT			
SUN			

Dates
____

Shopping List

Foods to Avoid

FOOD TRACKER JOURNAL

	BREAKFAST	LUNCH	DINNER
MON			
TUE			
WED			
THU			
FRI			
SAT			
SUN			

Dates

Shopping List

Foods to Avoid

FOOD TRACKER JOURNAL

	BREAKFAST	LUNCH	DINNER
MON			
TUE			
WED			
THU			
FRI			
SAT			
SUN			

Dates
____

Shopping List

Foods to Avoid

FOOD TRACKER JOURNAL

Dates

Shopping List

Foods to Avoid

	BREAKFAST	LUNCH	DINNER
MON			
TUE			
WED			
THU			
FRI			
SAT			
SUN			

Scan the QR code below to get a surprise bonus!

If you would love to have a one-on-one consultation session with Dr. Kelly Haaland, kindly reach out to us at kellyhaaland2@gmail.com.